PRACTICAL MR PHYSICS

PRACTICAL MR PHYSICS

AND CASE FILE OF MR ARTIFACTS AND PITFALLS

Alexander C. Mamourian, MD

Associate Professor of Radiology

Division of Neuroradiology

University of Pennsylvania

Philadelphia, Pennsylvania

OXFORD

UNIVERSITY PRESS

2010

OXFORD

UNIVERSITY PRESS

Oxford University Press, Inc. publishes works that further
Oxford University's objective of excellence
in research, scholarship and education.

Oxford New York
Auckland Cape Town Dar es Salaam Hong Kong Karachi
Kuala Lumpur Madrid Melbourne Mexico City Nairobi
New Delhi Shanghai Taipei Toronto

With offices in
Argentina Austria Brazil Chile Czech Republic France Greece
Guatemala Hungary Italy Japan Poland Portugal Singapore
South Korea Switzerland Thailand Turkey Ukraine Vietnam

Published by Oxford University Press Inc.
198 Madison Avenue, New York, New York 10016
www.oup.com

Oxford is a registered trademark of Oxford University Press

First published 2010

Library of Congress Cataloging-in-Publication Data
Mamourian, Alexander C.
Practical MR physics: And case file of MR artifacts and pitfalls / Alexander C. Mamourian.
p. ; cm.
Includes bibliographical references and index.
ISBN 978-0-19-537281-6
1. Medical physics. 2. Magnetic resonance imaging. 3. Nuclear magnetic resonance.
I. Title. [DNLM: 1. Magnetic Resonance Imaging—Case Reports. 2. Magnetic Resonance
Imaging—Problems and Exercises. 3. Image Interpretation, Computer-Assisted—Case Reports.
4. Image Interpretation, Computer-Assisted—Problems and Exercises. WN 18.2 M265p 2010]
R895.M26 2010
616.07'548—dc22
2009030871

All photographs by Alexander C. Mamourian.

1 3 5 7 9 8 6 4 2
Printed in the United States of America
on acid-free paper

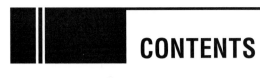

CONTENTS

PREFACE

When I filled out my application for a fellowship in MR imaging at the University of Pennsylvania 25 years ago, I was required to write an essay. I included in mine, at the urging of my sister Alicia, a plan to write a book about MR physics. I was never sure of whether it was because of, or in spite of, that essay the department chairman, Dr. Stanley Baum, accepted me for the fellowship but told me during my interview that this was among the most naive ideas he had ever heard from a prospective fellow. There was some truth to that since I was one year out of my residency training. It seems like a better idea now.

While MR physics has never been an easy subject to master, the bar is higher than ever since MR imaging techniques have become more complex. I suspect that many trainees have given up altogether and treat MR with due respect but at arms length, much as I treat my car's engine. Still, it is helpful to have some understanding of MR physics so that you can suggest ways to improve image quality and avoid mistaking common artifacts for disease.

I am not a physicist; this will prove to be a good thing for some readers and disappointing for others. Magnetic resonance imaging has been my professional focus for many years, however, and I hope you will find the explanations and analogies drawn from that experience clear and helpful. This book is not intended to replace the many fine books that focus on MR physics. While the basics of MR physics are included in Chapter 1, my goal is to use case material to illustrate how those principles will help you to identify and understand common artifacts. After reading this book, you will be better prepared to understand more advanced MR techniques as well.

The book is divided into four parts: (1) an overview of MR physics, (2) common MR artifacts, (3) common MR pitfalls, and (4) challenging cases. There are several ways you can use the book. For most readers who want to learn more about MR imaging, cover to cover will do best. You will also find in the book links to five instructional videos on the web that were created to complement this text. I encourage you to view them since the selected topics, such as the motion of precession, are easier to demonstrate than explain. If you are comfortable with the physics, a review of the artifacts and pitfalls should sharpen your imaging skills and will provide a refresher on MR physics. The answer for each case will be defined by a box, usually at the bottom of the page, so avert your gaze until you are ready for it. If you are an experienced imager but happen to encounter what you think is an artifact while you are reviewing clinical MR images, you can use the index in this book to investigate that topic. All readers should try to solve the puzzler cases either before or after reading the book, but the answers will surely come more easily afterward. It is my hope that this book proves to be valuable to you and, in that way, helpful to your patients.

ACKNOWLEDGMENTS

I am grateful for the time with my grandfather Garabed, who provided the groundwork; my parents, Marcus and Maritza, for helping me find my way; my sister Alicia, especially for drafting that essay; and my children, Ani, Molly, Liz, and Marcus, for giving me all the joyful reasons. To my wife Pam, words cannot express the depth of my gratitude for surely without you this book would have remained an unfulfilled promise.

I also want to thank the many gifted MR technologists I have worked with over the years, with special thanks to Swapan Sen, Chris Harris, Sharon Hurst, Bob Ferranti, Shreve Soule, and Theresa Haron, Theresa for both her competence and her keen eye.

My sincere thanks go to Andrea Seils at Oxford University Press for believing in this project, Josef Debbins, PhD, at the Barrow Institute, for keeping me true to the facts and guiding me to a better understanding of phase encoding, and to Doug Goodwin, MD, at Dartmouth-Hitchcock Medical Center for providing these exquisite musculoskeletal cases.

Finally, my eternal gratitude to Dr. Robert Spetzler and the NICU nursing staff at the Barrow Institute for giving me a second chance and inspiring me to write this book.

1 MR PHYSICS

The detailed images we can create with a magnetic resonance (MR) scanner using magnets, wires, and electricity are just as magical as X-ray images were for a previous generation. Unlike X-rays, however, MR imaging was not the result of a single moment of discovery. It represents the convergence of discoveries in the fields of physics, chemistry, and mathematics that occurred over the course of nearly 200 years.

In fact, it is hard to establish a single date for the beginning of the story of MR imaging once we acknowledge that the permanent magnets found in compasses have been used by sailors for over 2000 years. Nevertheless, a good starting point is that moment in 1820 when Hans Christian Oersted noticed, during a demonstration of electricity, that the needle of a nearby compass jumped when he attached a wire loop to a battery (Figure 1.1). This was the first reported evidence that these two powerful forces were linked. A decade would go by before Michael Faraday demonstrated the reciprocal effect of magnetic induction when he found that he could generate electrical current in a wire simply by moving a magnet back and forth in its vicinity (YouTube[1] video "Electricity MRphysics PennPhysics"). Throughout this overview of MR physics, you must always keep this interaction between magnetism and electricity in mind to understand how MR images are created.

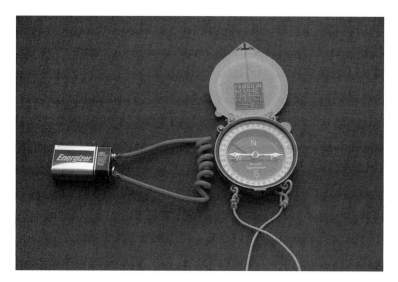

Figure 1.1 This arrangement of a battery, wire, and compass can be used to demonstrate the interaction of magnetism and electricity.

---

1 YouTube video "Electricity MRphysics": http://www.youtube.com/watch?v=zVz1MGSTLzQ.

Magnets

Strong magnets are an essential component of all MR scanners, and in the decades since the introduction of clinical MR, all three types of magnets, i.e., permanent, resistive, and superconducting, have been used for imaging. There have even been reports of imaging using the Earth's magnetic field, but this is closer to a parlor trick. Current medical imaging depends on magnets thousands of times more powerful, and the trends in scanner technology suggest that bigger is better. The reason such powerful magnets are utilized for MR imaging is that they are necessary to align the nuclei of hydrogen, which themselves behave like small magnets, and the stronger the magnet, the larger the effect on these atomic magnets.

Permanent magnets, which can be as humble as iron ore, have a very special property called *ferromagnetism*. Iron will spontaneously form small, discrete regions, called *domains*, where the magnetic poles of iron atoms fall into uniform alignment. The larger the domain, the stronger the magnetic field, with the logical extreme of having all the atoms forming a single domain. If iron is exposed to an extrinsic magnetic field, the small domains can coalesce, increasing their size and therefore their magnetic force, and will then stay that way. This explains why a screwdriver that may have been in use for years will suddenly start to pick up loose screws near its tip.

The formation of domains is temperature dependent, and they disappear above a specific temperature called the *Curie point,* named after Pierre Curie.[2] Iron, at a temperature above its Curie point, becomes paramagnetic, but as it cools, domains will form spontaneously; this makes iron unique and explains its natural ferromagnetic properties. Other, more exotic elements, like neodymium and boron, can be combined with iron to create powerful permanent magnets for applications as ubiquitous as the speakers inside tiny headphones. In all variations, the principle of innumerable small, atom-sized magnetic fields aligned to form a much larger one remains the same. The term *ferromagnetism* indicates that the magnetic property is intrinsic to the material. In contrast, the term *paramagnetism* is used to describe the transient alignment within an external magnetic field that is quickly lost once that extrinsic magnetic field is removed.

The appeal of these permanent magnets for imaging is obvious since they require no electrical current and provide their own magnetic shielding. The large magnetic fields created by the magnets used for medical imaging may extend far beyond the magnet. These peripheral magnetic fields need to be constrained because of rules and reasonable concerns about unwanted interactions with medical devices, such as pacemakers, when the field extends beyond the scanner room (YouTube[3] video "Fringe Field MRphysics"). This *fringe field* may not exceed 5G in hallways and public spaces like stairwells or corridors. Large plates of iron or steel can be used for *shielding* of electromagnets to contain their fringe field within the confines of a small room, but permanent magnets do not require this modification (Figure 1.2).

---

2 Pierre Curie was a professor of physics at the Sorbonne in Paris and he was married to Marie. He and Marie together were awarded one-half of the Nobel Prize in 1903 for their studies of spontaneous radiation, but his own early investigations concerned piezoelectricity and magnetism. The name *Curie point* acknowledges his discovery of this phenomenon as well. At the peak of his career, and just three years after he received the Nobel Prize, Pierre Curie was killed by a horse-drawn carriage as he crossed a street in Paris. This death, from a modern perspective, seems a remarkable intersection of the future and the past.
3 YouTube video "Fringe Field MRphysics": http://www.youtube.com/watch?v=8qFeUUegfII.

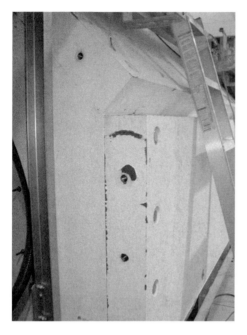

Figure 1.2 These large iron blocks are positioned within the housing of a superconducting magnet to make the magnetic field more compact. This allows the MR scanner to be placed in a room that may have formerly housed a CT scanner because the fringe field is now smaller.

The high initial acquisition cost of a permanent magnet for an MR scanner should be considered in light of potential savings in shielding, *cyrogens* (liquid gases), and electricity. While permanent magnets excel for some specialized applications like extremity imaging, they are limited for general medical imaging because of their weight, sensitivity to temperature change, and limits to field strength compared with their electromagnet relatives. For this reason, most manufacturers have turned to electromagnets.

The principle of all electromagnets, both superconducting and resistive, is that electricity flowing in a wire, as noted long ago by Oersted, can create a small magnetic field. This magnetic field can then be amplified by winding the wire around an iron core to form a useful electromagnet.

One essential difference between permanent magnets and electromagnets is that the latter can be switched on or off as needed. This is analogous to the difference between a horse and a car; no matter what the circumstances, only the car can be turned off. Movie fans may recall the large junkyard electromagnet that provided some dramatic effect in the James Bond movie *Goldfinger* when it was used to lift a neatly crushed Lincoln automobile into the air. After the metal cube was suspended for a moment, the electromagnet was turned off, dropping the block onto the bed of a waiting pickup truck. Smaller, and hopefully less dramatic, electromagnets can be found throughout our lives. One that is taken for granted almost daily is the automobile starter. It uses electric current from the battery to energize an electric motor in order to turn the engine over. The ability to turn electromagnets on and off makes them ideal for their role in MR scanners by creating the transient gradient fields used to modify the strong magnetic field.

While an iron core increases the field strength of an electromagnet, clinical magnets must have an *air core* in order to allow space for the patient in the center. The early scanners used field strengths of about 0.15 tesla (T), which seemed remarkably strong at the time but had only one-tenth the strength of the magnetic field used for routine MR imaging today. These early resistive scanners required a continuous supply of electrical current to create a strong magnetic field and, because of the property of electrical resistance, in the process created a considerable amount of heat. This unwanted by-product (remember that electrical resistance is the property that makes toasters and waffle irons hot) had to be removed in order to provide stability to the magnetic field. This was usually accomplished by cooling the magnet with water using a circulator and a radiator, much like the arrangement in a water-cooled car engine. There was also a tendency for the field to drift with temperature variations in the chilled water. The inherent instability and limited field strength of these early scanners, not to mention the high electricity bills, contributed to their surprisingly rapid replacement with super-conducting units.

Superconduction describes the unusual state of electrical current without any loss from resistance. This phenomenon was recognized in 1911 by Heike Kamerlingh Onnes, who discovered that the element mercury, cooled by liquid helium to nearly the temperature at which atomic motion stops (-459°F), loses any resistance to electrical current.[4] While based on the same fundamental principle as other electromagnets, superconducting magnets can achieve higher magnetic field strengths with-out the power demands or heating common to all resistive magnets. The wire used in these super-conducting electromagnets is made of an alloy of niobium and titanium interwoven in a complex arrangement with a conventional copper conductor and covered by a thin insulator. This highly specialized wire is necessary because the superconducting wire alone is not sufficient to handle the electrical current in the event of a sudden loss of cooling.

The magnet's design and construction also require a considerable degree of sophistication. The wraps of superconducting wire must stay in place as the magnet is energized, and the layers of insu-lation and copper must be thin enough to allow close proximity of the loops of wire while being, at the same time, sufficient in thickness for their tasks. Finally, the magnetic field must be both strong and uniform, a condition described as *homogeneity*. Some minor imperfections in the field can be corrected using *shim coils*. These are small electromagnets within the larger magnet that can be energized as needed. The wire is finally bathed in liquid helium to create the unique state of super-conduction (Figure 1.3).[5]

---

4 It is no coincidence that Onnes was also the first to generate liquid helium (1908). He received the Nobel Prize for his investigations into this realm of the supercold in 1913.

5 The dewar container seen in Figure 1.3 is named for Sir James Dewar, who studied liquid gases at the turn of the twentieth century. A dewar flask, strictly speaking, is a double-walled glass container that uses an intervening vacuum and a metal coating to provide extreme thermal isolation. While initially designed for the containment of supercold liquid gases, it proved excellent for keeping coffee warm as well and is now produced commercially and sold as the thermos bottle. As the wonderful rhetorical question goes, "It keeps cold things cold and hot things hot. How does it know?" Sir James Dewar, together with Sir Frederick Abel, also invented cordite, which was used as a powerful explosive and propellant for firearms throughout the British Empire.

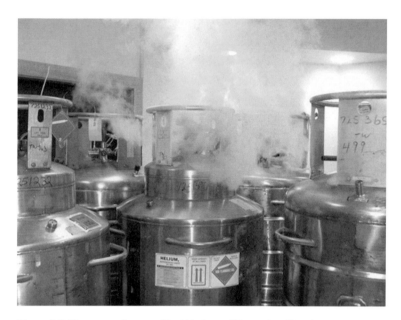

Figure 1.3 These many Dewars of liquid helium will be used to fill up the superconducting magnet of a 1.5 T MR scanner.

At the time of the introduction of these large superconducting magnets, there were some naysayers who doubted that these technological wonders could be managed in the general medical environment. History shows that their reservations were unfounded. These complex, powerful magnets make up the largest and in some ways the most important component of any MR scanner.

Magnetic fields are measured using the standard unit *gauss* (G), named after the mathematician Carl Friedrich Gauss. The most familiar and ubiquitous magnetic field we experience, the Earth's, measures about 0.5 G, while most refrigerator magnets fall in the 500–1000 G range. Because of their very strong magnetic fields, medical magnets are usually measured using a larger unit, much like pounds and tons, called a *tesla* (T), with 1.0 T equal to 10,000 G.[6]

Recently, clinical scanners using magnets of 3.0 T and research scanners with even stronger magnets have become commonplace. While there are some theoretical and practical limitations to medical imaging at 3.0 T, the motivation behind this migration to higher field strengths is to maximize the signal by recruiting a larger proportion of the available hydrogen nuclei in the body for imaging. The improvement in the signal-to-noise ratio that follows can in principle be used to provide some combination of better resolution, faster imaging, or thinner sections. There is a price to be paid, and not just financially, for these larger magnets. With the increase in magnetic

6 While Nicola Tesla was a brilliant inventor in his own right, and a contemporary of Thomas Edison, he never enjoyed the same recognition as Edison. Tesla surpassed Edison in the end, however, with his prediction that alternating current would prove to be better for local power delivery than Edison's choice of direct current.

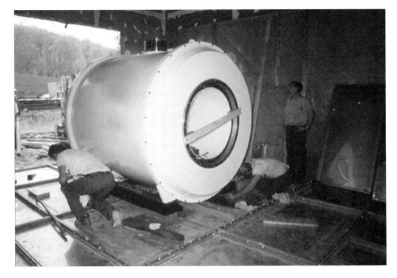

Figure 1.4 This is a picture of the 1.5 T superconducting magnet that was installed at Hershey-Penn State University Medical Center in 1985. This cylinder contains the superconducting wire and functions like a giant Dewar by providing thermal insulation for the liquid gases. Note the metal plates on the wall and floor that provide RF shielding for the scanner. This isolates the scanner from intruding radio waves that may be detected by the sensitive antenna and projected onto the image.

field strength comes greater power deposition in the body of the patient, decreased T1 contrast, increased risk from metal in the room, and larger chemical shift effects. For some applications, however, like magnetic resonance angiography (MRA) or detailed structural imaging, the trade-off appears to be acceptable.

A superconducting magnet, once energized with electrical power, requires no additional current. For this reason, a superconducting scanner behaves more like a permanent magnet than an electro-magnet because it is *always on*. This is also unlike other medical imaging devices that may have an outwardly similar appearance, like computed tomography (CT) scanners, but can be turned off at night.

While the notion of a powerful field with no power costs is very attractive, the energy cost of superconduction comes with the replenishment of liquid helium. This supercold liquid surrounds the wire within a strongly insulated container (Figure 1.4) but boils off continually in spite of its high degree of thermal isolation. Replacing the liquid gas requires access to this container through a special apparatus called a *cold head*, installed at the top of the scanner's magnet (Figure 1.5). The time between helium refills can be extended with the use of a helium pump to regenerate the liquid gas. It is this device that provides that incessant "puckata-puckata" sound that is always audible, even when the scanner is not being used for imaging.

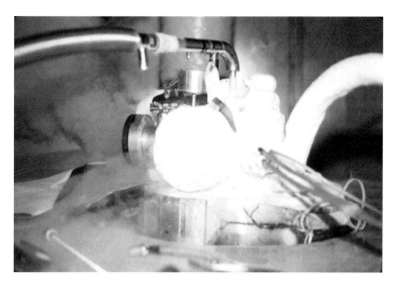

Figure 1.5 Frost forms on the *cold head* at the top of the MR scanner where moisture in the air freezes as it meets the extreme cold due to the liquid helium within. This device provides access to the magnet for the helium refills.

Precession

Magnetic resonance imaging is possible only because hydrogen is intrinsically magnetic and, at the same time, abundant in the human body. The magnetic properties of hydrogen give it polarity, i.e., a north pole and a south pole like those of the Earth or any bar magnet. And, as we have come to expect with a compass needle, these magnetic poles of the hydrogen atom tend to align when they are exposed to the strong external magnetic field of the MR scanner.

The nucleus of a hydrogen atom consists of a single positively charged proton that, as predicted by Pauli in 1924, is constantly spinning. This spin of an electrically charged particle creates a very weak magnetic field that forms, in principle, much like the magnetic field created by moving charges in a wire (see the discussion on page 2). While the composite magnetic field of even hundreds of hydrogen nuclei would be too small to detect, the magnetic field created by the alignment of a small fraction of the trillions of hydrogen nuclei in the human body becomes sufficient to be measured indirectly.

This property of spin not only contributes to the magnetic field of protons, it also gives hydrogen protons the quality of *angular momentum*. Common to moving things, with momentum comes an aversion to change. In the special case of angular momentum, a force on the axis of spin creates torque and movement occurs, improbably, in the direction of the torque that is perpendicular to the displacing force. This results in a special type of movement in a spinning object called *precession*. This is easier to picture with familiar objects than to explain, so consider the toy top or gyroscope (YouTube[7] video "Precession MRphysics").

The initial spin gives the top a very high rotational frequency along its long axis. As this axis is pulled down by gravity, the top demonstrates a lazy, large rotational motion around the bottom pin.

7 YouTube video "Precession MRphysics": http://www.youtube.com/watch?v=V8F-KLhrtTE.

This second rotational movement is precession. It is important to consider, and is not at all obvious, that the frequency of this precession is directly proportional to the strength of the displacing force. In the case of the top, the displacing force is gravity, so we should expect that the frequency of precession of the top would be lower on the Moon and higher on Jupiter because of their respectively lower and higher gravitational attraction compared with that of the Earth.

We can think of the spinning hydrogen nucleus in the same way as the top, but the displacing force, instead of gravity, is the scanner magnet. And, just like the effect of gravity on the top, the stronger the magnetic field, the higher the frequency of precession. This relationship was reported by Sir Joseph Larmor, who predicted that the exact frequency of nuclear precession could be calculated as the product of the strength of the magnetic field experienced by the hydrogen nuclei and a "gyro-magnetic constant" specific for the nucleus of interest. The symbolic representation of this relationship is called the *Larmor equation*.

$$\omega_0 = \gamma \, \mathbf{B}_0$$

ω_0 = frequency of precession
γ = gyro-magnetic constant specific for the atom
$\mathbf{B}_0$ = the magnetic field

Scanners can be described by their magnetic field strength or by the frequency of precession of the hydrogen nuclei within the magnet. For example, a 1.0 T scanner can be described as a 42 MHz scanner and a 1.5 T scanner as a 63 MHz scanner based on the *Larmor frequency* of hydrogen at each field strength. This tightly linked relationship of field strength and frequency is essential to for your understanding of MR physics and frequency encoding in particular.

Resonance

Resonance: A vibration of large amplitude in a mechanical or electrical system caused by a relatively small periodic stimulus of the same or nearly the same period as the natural vibration period of the system.

Merriam-Webster Online Dictionary

You need look no further than a backyard swing set to find an everyday example of resonance (YouTube[8] video "Resonance MRphysics"). We intuitively recognize that lifting the passenger on the swing higher and higher requires precise timing of the push. At the same time, we are aware that the incremental force of the push is trivial compared with the energy that would be required to toss the passenger into the air with one push. Resonance describes this process of applying small but optimally timed pushes that match the natural frequency of the swing.

We pick up the story of MR imaging again with the discovery of nuclear magnetic resonance (NMR) by Isidor Isaac Rabi.[9] Using a device that created a narrow stream of lithium chloride molecules, first developed by Otto Stern and Walter Gerlach, Rabi found a remarkable interaction of

8 YouTube video "Resonance MRphysics": http://www.youtube.com/watch?v=tpl2skw0TZ4.
9 Rabi is an inspiring example of a somewhat lackluster young student who developed into a brilliant researcher. He is also credited for his work in the years just before receiving the Nobel Prize for the development of radar, which proved to be critical to the Allies' victory in World War II. While Rabi's insights laid the groundwork for NMR and MR imaging, strangely he has not received widespread recognition in the medical community.

these charged particles with radio waves and a magnetic field. On the basis of these experiments, he received a Nobel Prize in 1944 for his discovery that the interaction of these charged molecules with the magnetic field and RF energy was due to nuclear resonance.

This principle, established in Rabi's physics laboratory, forms the basis for MR imaging, but four decades would pass before the last pieces of that puzzle would fall into place. In the MR scanner, the magnetic polarity of the many hydrogen nuclei (protons) becomes aligned to some degree by the strong external magnetic field inside the bore of the scanner. However, these nuclei will not just snap into place inside the scanner, all pointing north and south like compass needles. Because of their angular momentum and the displacing force of the magnet, these hydrogen nuclei will precess at a frequency predicted by the Larmor equation. While they are stationary but precessing at the same time, you can think of them like trout swimming in place in a stream. While the trout stay roughly aligned with the current, they are always moving, albeit in one preferred location.

While in practice we use an RF pulse to add additional energy to this natural movement of the hydrogen nuclei, it may be easier to picture the resonant force as a magnet moving on a track around the bore of the magnet. Just like the pushing of a swing, the pace of this smaller magnet must match precisely the natural frequency of the hydrogen precession in order to satisfy the necessary conditions for resonance. Not all but some significant fraction of the many trillions of hydrogen spins will be captured by the field of this moving magnet. As the nuclei become energized by this attraction, their magnetic axis will begin to point away from the long axis of the scanner bore and toward this imaginary magnet on the track until they point perpendicular to the large scanner magnet. At that moment, the individual magnetic poles of all these protons will also be pointing in the same direction, i.e., toward the moving magnet, which maximizes the strength of their composite field. The RF transmitter effectively acts the same way, imparting energy to the ordered but precessing hydrogen nuclei. The hydrogen protons, with their magnetic poles pointing in the same direction but perpendicular to the strong field, can be described as having experienced a 90 degree RF pulse and are now in coherent phase.

I must warn you to avoid unclear thinking due to mixing the image of single hydrogen spins with the composite magnetic field that reflects the sum of many of these spins. At this point, let's change our focus; let's stop thinking about single hydrogen protons and think instead of the net force created by the sum of many individual spins. You can now think of this composite field as a single spinning bar magnet pointing in the direction perpendicular to the long axis of the scanner bore (Figure 1.6), and we know that a moving magnetic field will induce an electrical current in a wire inside the scanner. We can call that wire an antenna and, using it, we can register a rising and falling electrical current as this bar magnet (composed of countless hydrogen nuclei) spins nearby. This waveform will have the same frequency as the hydrogen Larmor frequency and an amplitude determined by the total number of hydrogen nuclei spinning together.

This is precisely how the NMR signal is detected and it represents the state of the art in 1952, the year that Felix Bloch and Edward Purcell received their Nobel Prizes for NMR spectroscopy. Their work brought this phenomenon of NMR out of the laboratory and to the level where it could be used as a laboratory tool for investigation of the composition of solids, liquids, and gases. While MR imaging almost always uses hydrogen nuclei, NMR can be used for a wide range of elements so long as their nuclei have an odd number of charges, such as phosphorus or sodium.

Chemists were entranced by this technique that allowed them to examine nondestructively small chemical samples using only their radio waves. Prior to the discovery of NMR, it was not so easy

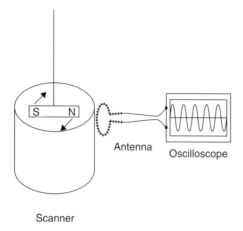

Antenna Oscilloscope

Scanner

Figure 1.6 The net magnetic force of the collectively aligned hydrogen nuclei after a 90 degree RF pulse acts very much like a spinning bar magnet. The reason we can recover signal from a human body comes back to the principle that a moving magnet will induce current in a nearby wire. This spinning magnet will then induce a fluctuating current in a nearby wire (antenna) as it spins towards, and then away from, the antenna. The frequency of the resulting wave can be predicted by the Larmor equation and is based on a gyromagnetic constant and the magnetic field strength the hydrogen spins experience.

to determine the constituents of chemical compounds and it usually involved some mix of torches, solvents, and crystals. What makes NMR so powerful is that the waveform recovered, and then converted to a spectrum, is altered by chemical bonds and other elements in the vicinity of the stimulated atom. To minimize confounding factors, great emphasis was placed on creating a completely homogeneous magnetic field. During the many years that scientists worked exclusively with NMR spectrometers, however, there were no recorded attempts to use it for imaging.

Imaging

The pieces were all in place at this point for the transition from NMR spectra to MR imaging. Diverging from the usual practice of studying chemical compounds with NMR spectrometers, Dr. Raymond Damadian used one to test his hypothesis that the NMR character of liver tumors differed in a predictable fashion from that of normal liver. His experimental proof opened the conceptual door to medical uses for NMR, and he reported the results of his research in the journal *Science* in 1971. Paul Lauterbur in 1973 reported in the journal *Nature* his novel technique for modifying NMR hardware in order to create images,[10] while Peter Mansfield, across the Atlantic, was developing pulse sequences that could be used for imaging. Just 10 years after the appearance of Dr. Lauterbur's paper in *Nature*, clinical MR scanners were being installed throughout the United States, but 20 years more would go by before the Nobel committee decided to award Lauterbur and Mansfield their prizes. It was in these early days of imaging that the terminology changed subtly from *nuclear magnetic resonance* to just *magnetic resonance*, with the thought that the *n* for *nuclear* in the name might be confused with *nuclear medicine* or alarming for some patients.

Dr. Lauterbur's innovation was to modify the strong NMR magnetic field in a uniform and predictable fashion using smaller magnets called *gradient coils*. With this addition, the magnetic field could then be varied from front to back, side to side, and top to bottom. Since we know that the

10 It is of some comfort to researchers everywhere that his paper, later ranked among the most significant scientific papers ever published, was initially rejected.

magnetic field strength predicts the frequency of precession (Larmor equation), and if we know where the field is stronger or weaker, we could in principle establish the location of the returning signal based on its frequency alone. This concept of modifying the magnetic field to establish the spatial location of the returning signal is basic to all MR imaging (Figure 1.7).

This notion of diagnostic MR imaging may seem mundane now, what with MR scanners in trucks and shopping malls, but it was remarkable at the time. It may also come as a surprise that the poor resolution of these early images, compared with the detailed images provided by the more mature technology of CT, led some imagers to downplay the impact of this new imaging tool when the first clinical scanners were introduced (Figure 1.8). Now let's consider exactly how one might use these magnetic gradients to make detailed images of the body. It is easier to explain localization of signal with a simpler object than the human body, so let's start by imaging some wine bottles in a wine rack (Figure 1.9). Let's see if we can use the MR scanner to determine which slots are empty and which slots are filled in a rack with three slots across and three side (3 × 3).

While imaging can be done by creating a "sweet spot" where resonance occurs, but nowhere else, and moving the rack around it, this approach is not practical. Nevertheless, it is effective and was used to create the first published human body image with MR. In all current clinical MR units, the images are created by using gradient coils that are turned on and off in a sequential pattern. The order and timing of their activation can be most easily depicted using a pulse sequence diagram with a different timeline for each piece of the scanner hardware. This is not much different from a musical score that a composer uses to indicate when the violins come in, the flutes drop out, and all the while the drums play on (Figure 1.10).

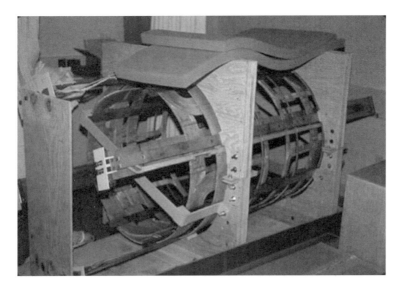

Figure 1.7 This is a photograph of a gradient coil assembly prior to installation in an early 1.5 T unit. (The wooden frame supports the coils in transit.) These electromagnets will be placed within the open center of the large superconducting magnet where they will surround the patient. The coils are energized in pairs so that the magnetic field inside the scanner bore may be modified in a roughly linear fashion from top to bottom, side to side, and head to toe.

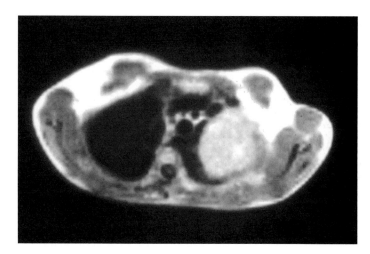

Figure 1.8 This axial MR scan of the chest was obtained in 1983 on an early 0.15 T resistive MR scanner at the University of Pennsylvania. While not up to the standards of current production MR scanners, it was remarkable at that time and still provided the diagnosis of a lung tumor in this patient. That early clinical scanner, however, provided only one slice at a time, placing a premium on the imager's knowledge of surface anatomy.

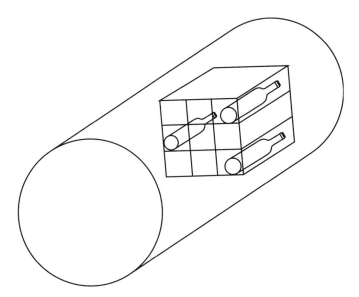

Figure 1.9 This drawing indicates the position of three bottles of wine that are arranged in a 9-slot wine rack (three by three) that resides inside the bore of an MR scanner.

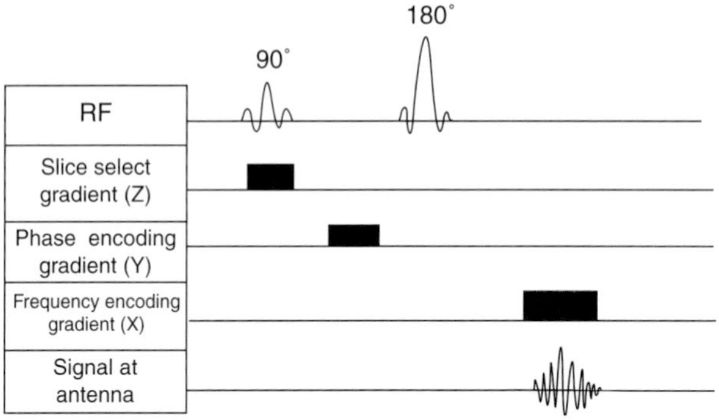

Figure 1.10 This is a much simplified pulse diagram for a spin echo MR scan. The different action lines can be thought of just like a music score that indicates when the different instruments come in, for how long, and at what volume. The bottom line indicates when the signal will be detected at the antenna in relation to the other actions.

Slice Selection

Using our wine rack example, we can take the first step toward spatial localization, called *slice selection*. Since most images for diagnosis are displayed like so many slices of bread, it is reasonable to acquire the information in the same fashion. It is worth noting that since this is done entirely with the use of electronic gradients and without any fixed hardware (like an X-ray tube spinning in a CT scanner), any and all planes of acquisition are possible in an MR scanner.

Let's position our wine rack inside the scanner so that the corks of the bottles are pointing away from us as we look inside the scanner bore. We will name the gradient that runs from the top to the bottom of the bottles the *Z gradient* direction. When this gradient is turned on, it modifies the previously uniform strong magnetic field so that it is now higher at the top of the bottles and lower at the bottoms. This leaves a band right in the middle where the hydrogen spins experience no more or less than the native strong magnetic field. It is fairly straightforward, then, to use the radiofrequency (RF) transmitter to impart energy at the frequency that matches the precession frequency of that band in order to move the hydrogen spins into the plane perpendicular to the scanner bore, called a *90 degree pulse*. While all the hydrogen spins inside the scanner will experience this same RF pulse, only those in that narrow slice will resonate with the RF pulse and absorb energy. In other parts of the rack, where the conditions for resonance are not fulfilled, those hydrogen nuclei become effectively invisible. In this fashion, we can get signal back from just one slice through the bottles at a level midway from the neck to the base.

This signal that we recover with the antenna tells us that there are some wine bottles in that slice, but it provides no information about their location. The amplitude of the returning wave tells us indirectly how many bottles are in the rack since more wine bottles mean more hydrogen nuclei and therefore more signal.

The electrical current or signal that registers at the antenna may be displayed as a waveform with a frequency and an amplitude. While it is simple to graph this signal with elapsed time on the horizontal axis and amplitude on the vertical axis, when multiple frequencies are mixed together, it is easier to understand when we *Fourier transform* this into a spectrum, i.e., a graph of amplitude on the vertical axis and frequency on the horizontal axis (Figure 1.11).

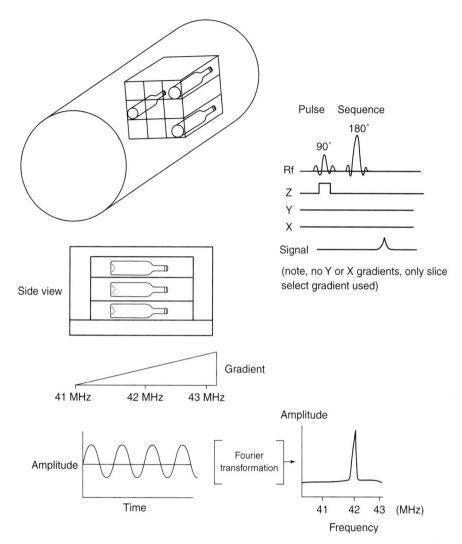

Side view

Gradient

41 MHz   42 MHz   43 MHz

Pulse   Sequence

180°

90°

Rf

Z

Y

X

Signal

(note, no Y or X gradients, only slice
select gradient used)

Amplitude

Amplitude

Time

Fourier
transformation

41   42   43   (MHz)

Frequency

Figure 1.11 This illustration demonstrates the aspects of slice selection. By applying a magnetic gradient that varies from the bottom to the top of the bottles, only one slice in the middle will be at the correct frequency for resonance with the RF energy. The pulse diagram shows that just one gradient, the Z or slice select, is used for this step. The waveform we recover with the antenna from the water (actually hydrogen nuclei in the wine) can be displayed as a waveform or, after Fourier transformation, a spectrum with amplitude on the vertical axis and frequency on the bottom. Note that only one frequency is present, at the Larmor frequency of water determined by the magnetic field (1.0 T).

Frequency Encoding

Now at least we have reduced the problem of assigning spatial location to the signal to only two directions, up or down and left or right. We can solve that problem using the two remaining gradient pairs. The left-right location can be determined by turning on the side-to-side gradient (X gradient) during the collection of the signal after the 90 degree pulse. By using a gradient pair to modify the strong magnetic field from side to side, the field becomes stronger on one side than the other. Since the frequency of precession is linked to field strength, and supposing that the field is now higher on the right than on the left, we would then know that any high-frequency signal we recover at the antenna comes from the right side of the scanner and the low-frequency signal comes from the left side. This assignment of spatial location based on frequency alone is called *frequency encoding*. You are already familiar with the concept of spatial location linked to frequency at a more intuitive level involving musical instruments. When you hear a low, rumbling note coming from a piano, you can envision that the player hit a key on the left side of the keyboard without actually seeing the keyboard. You also know, when figuring out how to play a song on the piano, that if the note you strike is too low, you will move to keys on your right, where the frequency of the notes is higher. This predictable spatial–frequency relationship between the keyboard and audible notes is a form of frequency encoding.

This process of frequency encoding brings us to Fourier transformation. This mathematical function is perhaps most easily understood using a biologic example. The function of the cochlea in the ear is to convert the multiple complex frequencies of sound waves that enter the ear canal into discrete neural signals that indicate which frequencies are represented. For example, the low-frequency sound of a tuba stimulates a specific part of the cochlea to provide electrical signals that then register in the cortex of the brain. This function of the cochlea allows us to recognize the unique sound of this and any other musical instrument. The conversion of sound into a signal with an amplitude that also indicates the volume of that sound captures the basic concept of the Fourier transformation.[11]

Using Fourier transformation, we can convert a complex signal composed of multiple frequencies, detected by the antenna, into its component frequencies, much as the ear and cochlea function together. Fourier transformation proves to be a critical process in MR image reconstruction to the point that the matrix choices we use for imaging (128, 256, 512) are dictated by the requirements of fast Fourier transformation (FFT).

---

11 This mathematical function is named for Joseph Fourier, and the story of his life may cause you to reconsider any stereotype you might have of a bookish mathematician. The 9th of 12 children who was orphaned at age 9, he nearly went to the guillotine for his role in the French Revolution, became a scientific advisor to Napoleon, and was for a time stranded in Egypt after the British admiral Horatio Nelson eviscerated the French navy. His mathematical work directed at calculating heat transfer proved to be ideal for MR image processing 150 years after he died. He is also credited with the observation that the atmosphere functions as a heat-retaining blanket around the Earth. His contributions are certainly in the forefront in this millennium.

By turning on this second gradient while we recover signal from the one slice through the middle of the bottles, instead of recovering a single frequency from the hydrogen protons at their Larmor frequency, multiple frequencies will be represented in the signal, depending on the location of the bottles. So, at this point, we should be able to figure out which columns (left, center, or right) in the rack have at least one bottle of wine. If there is more than one bottle in any column, we should be able to guess this because the signal at that frequency will have increased amplitude, since there will be more hydrogen protons producing the signal (Figure 1.12). Now we have two dimensions of signal assignment, and we will leave the third coordinate to the technique of *phase encoding*.

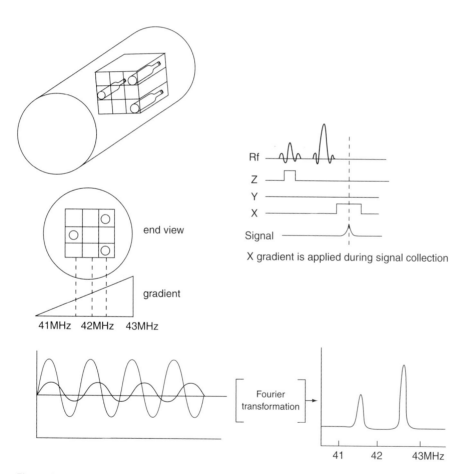

Figure 1.12 In this illustration we see the aspects of frequency selection. The gradient field is applied from side to side so that the wine bottles on your right will experience a stronger magnetic field than those on your left. Now, instead of recovering signal at just one frequency at the antenna, we see two different waveforms since the hydrogen nuclei in the two bottles on your right provide signal with both a higher frequency and amplitude since there are more hydrogens with two bottles. After the Fourier transform of the recovered signal, note these two peaks depict those differences in frequency and amplitude of signal.

Phase Encoding Explained

How can we use the phase of the returning signal to indicate if the bottles in any column are at the top, bottom, or middle of that column? And what is phase anyway?

Phase encoding is not a single-step localization process like the first two. It also is the most difficult to explain because it is more of a mathematical process than an intuitive concept. But, rather than say that "something really amazing happens," let's examine it carefully since some basic understanding of this principle will help you to better understand the artifacts that follow. It is also helpful to consider at the outset that frequency and phase can be considered interchangeable. When we see a waveform moving up and down along the time axis, this same information can be represented by a measure of its relative phase at specific points in time. This is somewhat analogous to the way music can be stored in an analog form that captures the wave itself (vinyl records) or by sampling that same wave and then storing it in a digital file (CDs). That later process is called *analog-to-digital conversion*, and the number of data points used to measure the sound waves reflects how accurately the sound will be reproduced. This principle of digital sampling of a sound waveform is essentially how music is stored as a digital file in your iPod.

It is worth pointing out again that at the moment the RF pulse is turned off, the energized hydrogen protons are not only rotating perpendicular to the large magnetic field, they are also pointing in exactly the same direction (*coherent phase*). *Phase* is the term used to describe the orientation of the magnetic axis of each hydrogen proton. When the hydrogen protons are considered as a population, and when the magnetic poles of these protons align, their net magnetic force is amplified. However, even when they are energized into the 90 degree plane, the loss of coherent phase among the protons will result in a lower net magnetic force.

When these hydrogen nuclei are considered as a population, there will be both constructive and destructive interactions due to phase on net magnetization For example, consider a single voxel where there are 1 million energized hydrogen spins all rotating in the transverse plane with coherent phase. In this circumstance, the net magnetic force, which will induce current in the antenna, will be quite large because the small magnetic field of each proton is reinforced by its 999,999 neighbors. This is reminiscent of the property of domains we reviewed in the discussion of permanent magnets. However, if the magnetic axes of these same protons are spread randomly in every direction, even though these protons are spinning in the transverse plane, their net magnetic force will be zero because of cancellation of this force. This happens because protons with opposite phase will cancel each other with respect to their composite or net magnetic field. This is also an illustration of the difference between the dynamics of a single hydrogen proton and that of a whole population.

When we turn the third (Y) gradient on in order to make the magnetic field stronger at the top than at the bottom of the columns, the frequency of precession of the hydrogen protons at the top of the column will become greater than the frequency of precession of the protons at the bottom. This also means that there will be a *phase shift* across the column as the protons speed up or slow down relative to the middle row, where the phase shift is zero. The moment the Y gradient is turned off, the hydrogen nuclei in each column will go back to spinning at the same frequency, but they retain the phase shift acquired while the Y gradient was on. The longer the Y gradient is left on, the larger this phase shift will be from the top to the bottom of the column.

The extent of this phase shift can be described in terms of the relative spread of the phase of individual protons from the top to the bottom, i.e., 90 degrees, 120 degrees, 180 degrees, and so on. If there is no shift at all, this is called the *coherent phase*. Using the gradient, the total spread of available phase shifts is 180 degrees to –180 degrees for a total of 360 degrees. Keep in mind that any phase shifts beyond 360 degrees will become ambiguous since 370 degrees would look the same as 10 degrees to the scanner, just as 0900 hours (military time) looks no different than 2100 on a wall clock.

If at this point we could determine the frequency and absolute phase shift of the signal arising from the protons that we recover at the antenna, we might have the information we need to create an image. Unfortunately, the problem of spatial location using phase encoding proves to be more difficult just because the scanner cannot determine phase directly. Because of the phase interactions of populations of hydrogen protons, however, phase can be measured indirectly, but it requires repeated applications of a varying Y gradient in order to decipher it.

Coming back to the wine rack in the scanner, since we know there are two bottles in the far right column and one in the far left column, we must now determine if they are at the top, middle, or bottom of the columns. To illustrate how this problem can be solved using phase information, let's illustrate the effects of phase change on net magnetization or signal using a belt and two clothespins. Each pin in this example will represent the phase of one of two hydrogen protons. If the belt is placed flat on a table and two pins are placed on the same side of the belt, that arrangement would resemble the state of phase coherence. In that condition, the magnetic fields of these two protons would add together nicely (Figure 1.13).

Now, let's twist the belt buckle one full turn, creating a 180 degree phase shift. If we look at the belt from the single view to replicate the limitations in measuring phase, we would see it as the "end-on" view in Figure 1.14. As you can see, with coherent phase, you cannot tell where the clips reside on the belt. However, with a 180 degree twist (phase shift) in the belt, things become clearer. In this simple example, if the clips point in opposite directions seen from our end-on view, then we could predict that they must be at opposite ends of the belt (Figure 1.15), and if they point in nearly the same direction, they must be very close together indeed.

The scanner, of course, has no end-on view, but it does measure signal amplitude. Consider what might happen to the amplitude of recovered signal at the antenna with these two extremes of phase shift. Coherent phase should produce maximum signal no matter where the bottles reside in the rack. The lowest signal amplitude, or even no signal at all, will be recovered using a 180 degree phase shift if the bottles in the rack are at the top and bottom slots due to cancellation of the opposite phase directions. If, on the other hand, the bottles are in adjacent racks, a small drop in signal will be evident after the 180 degree phase shift. This is how signal intensity alterations after these known phase shifts provide some degree of spatial information. Multiple phase shifts with collection of accompanying signal will be required to determine the exact spatial location of the returning signal, however.

In practice, this requires varying the Y gradient for every row of information in the phase direction of the matrix. Think of expanding this problem of spatial localization from finding three bottles in a wine rack with nine possible slots to an image with a matrix of 512 × 512 and subtle shadings of signal, and you can better appreciate the calculations and complexities involved in applying this concept of phase encoding to MR imaging (Figure 1.16).

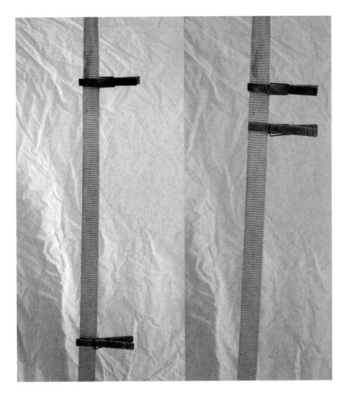

Figure 1.13 This photograph of two clothes pins on a belt are meant to illustrate two individual hydrogen protons with coherent phase, rotating at the same frequency, but at different locations in the phase direction. If we were to briefly apply a magnetic gradient from top to bottom the clips on each belt would experience a slightly different magnetic field strength that would then alter their rotational frequency. The greater the distance between the clips, or hydrogen spins, the larger the difference in their frequencies.

Coherent phase

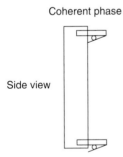

Side view

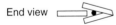

End view

Figure 1.14

180 phase shift

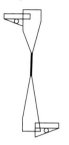

  Figure 1.15

Phase Encoding

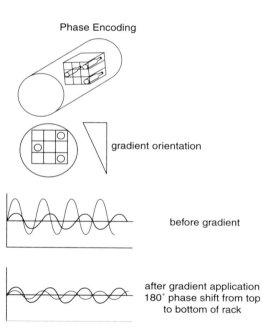

gradient orientation

before gradient

after gradient application
180° phase shift from top
to bottom of rack

Figure 1.16 In this illustration we see the Y gradient applied so that the magnetic field is briefly higher at the top than at the bottom of the column. This will make the protons at the top precess faster than those at the bottom and, depending on how long or how strongly the gradient is applied, different magnitudes of phase shift can be created. Before the application of the 180 degree phase shift, and after application of the frequency (side to side gradient), we see the two waveforms of different amplitude and frequency shown in figure 12. When the same frequency gradient is applied after a 180 degree shift of the vertical columns of spins, notice how the amplitude of the higher frequency signal is diminished. This is due to phase cancellation that reflects indirectly that there must be a bottle at the top and bottom of that particular frequency column. In this fashion, by varying the phase gradient and recording the changes in the returning signal, the location of the bottles (or really spins) can then be determined in each vertical columns.

Phase and Frequency

Magnetic resonance scanners use a sophisticated mathematical tool called *two-dimensional (2D) Fourier transformation* to handle this complex problem. However, the data points can't be entered for this calculation as "frequency," so the recovered signal must be described by just its *magnitude* and *phase*. Magnitude we understand as the amplitude or strength of the signal we recover at the antenna. But rather than describe the returning signal by its frequency, we can use the relative phase of the returning waveform.

Returning to frequency encoding, we used the X gradient to modify the strong magnetic field of the scanner from side to side. This will result in a range of frequencies that we recover at the antenna after the 90 degree pulse, and this range encodes spatial location. This frequency information can be expressed by a measurement of relative phase. For example, if we use 42 MHz as our reference frequency for a 1.0 T scanner, since that is the Larmor frequency of hydrogen at that field strength, we can describe the returning signal at that frequency as having zero phase shift. If we then compare that to signal a 43 MHz signal and measure from a point where they simultaneously cross the time axis, then we can see that the 43 MHz wave has a relative phase difference compared with the 42 MHz reference signal because it is cycling faster (Figure 1.17). The applied X gradient is adjusted to match the field of view in order to shift the frequencies from left to right in such a way that the phase shifts of the outermost voxels are –180 degrees (left) and 180 degrees (right) relative to zero phase (at the center). This characterization of the frequency of the returning signal by its magnitude and relative phase is necessary to meet the requirements of Fourier transformation.

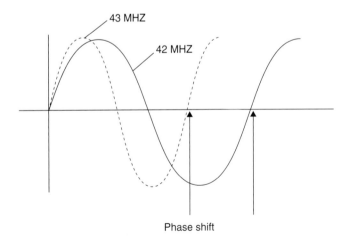

43 MHZ

42 MHZ

Phase shift

Figure 1.17 These two waveforms differ in frequency. While this difference can be expressed as a 1 MHz difference, it can also be expressed by the measure of their relative phase shift.

K-Space

This magnitude and phase information, which together are called a *complex number*, must be stored in the computer's memory as it is collected. This conceptual storage space is called *k-space*, and because each number contains both magnitude and phase information, there must be a "double cubby" in k-space to store each part. In addition, there must be one pair of numbers for each voxel that we will eventually reconstruct in the X direction. In fact, k-space would appear at first glance to have the right number of cubbies when measured from side to side as well as from top to bottom as the final image, so it would be quite logical to think that this data arrangement corresponds to the final image, but this would be wrong. The rows in k-space do not provide information about a corresponding line in the final image like the lines on an old-fashioned cathode ray TV screen. Rather, each point in k-space represents the information that is collected from all the voxels in the image. Remember that the antenna "hears" the returning signal from every point in the slice at once. This may seem a bit mind-boggling, but once we have collected all of the data necessary to fill k-space, we can then use the Fourier transform to sort everything out and take us right back to image space where we can feel more comfortable.

Each line of the information we will store in k-space is acquired after a slight alteration in the Y gradient that must applied before the signal collection. Since we want the phase to vary from −180 to 180 from the bottom to the top of k-space, just as we established for left to right, the bottommost line will have the strongest gradient force to create the −180 phase. Then, as each echo is acquired (one echo for each time to repetition), the strength of the gradient will be decreased slightly, becoming weaker and weaker as we fill the lower half of k-space. When we cross the center of k-space, there is no Y gradient because we want the center line to have *zero* phase shift. Then we will continue to increase the gradient in the opposite direction for each echo collected until we reach the top, where the strongest gradient effect will induce a +180 phase for the final signal collection. Each variation in the Y gradient will result in an alteration of the strength of the signal at each frequency because of constructive or destructive phase interactions. This varying interaction encodes spatial information just like twisting our belt to find the clothespins.

Since the center line of k-space (zero phase shift) represents signal at maximum, the nearby small phase shifts will incur some small degree of signal loss while the larger phase shifts have considerably more. If you think about it, while a zero phase shift has the most signal, it also has the least amount of spatial information. By contrast, the top and bottom rows of k-space where the phase shifts are largest and the signal intensity is lowest contain much more spatial information. As a result of this arrangement, the center portion of k-space is rich with image contrast information, while the periphery contains most of the detail information.

In this way, we satisfy the FFT condition by filling k-space so that there is a −180 to +180 phase shift in each direction. At this point, we simply hand this complex valued (magnitude and phase) k-space over to the computer (now we are back to "something amazing happens") and ask it to perform the Fourier transform in two dimensions.

"Two-dimensional transformation?" you may be thinking. You can better understand this notion by following this line of reasoning. First, you need to accept the idea that we can determine location in one direction based on frequency alone (think of the piano keyboard). Then, you should recognize that the frequency of a wave can also be expressed in terms of its phase, and it is this phase information that is registered in k-space. So, since k-space is symmetric and since we know the phase information in every point of k-space, the 2D Fourier transformation extracts a frequency for every spatial point using that phase information in both directions. This calculation is based on the *rate of change* of phase. If you stop to think about it, a high-frequency waveform can be described as having a high rate of phase change, while a low-frequency waveform has a low rate of phase change. So, as far as the 2D FFT is concerned, there is no difference in the calculation of frequency from side to side or top to bottom.

The result of this 2D Fourier transformation is in fact a complex image that contains both magnitude and phase information. We typically discard the phase information, and use the magnitude information as the basis for assigning to each pixel a dark or bright value. This, of course, becomes what we then call an *MR image*.

K-Space Applications

While the concept of k-space may seem abstract (because it is), it may be helpful to consider how the assignment of data to k-space can be used to explain both how the fast spin echo (FSE) sequence is acquired and the resulting quality of the images. This should help to explain why FSE T2-weighted imaging (T2WI) has replaced conventional spin echo imaging and, indirectly, why fluid-attenuated inversion recovery (FLAIR) has replaced the FSE proton density sequence for routine brain imaging.

At one time, MR scans were obtained using what we now call *conventional spin echo imaging*. With this technique, one line of k-space was filled after each variation of the phase gradient and a discrete 90 degree pulse was necessary for each application of the phase gradient. Using this approach, the total scan time was calculated by multiplying the time to repetition (TR) x the number of phase encoding steps x the number of acquisitions. Scans with a long TR or high matrix could take quite a while to complete. For example, a FLAIR scan using a TR of 10,000 msec, a 256×512 matrix, and 2 NEX would take 10 seconds $\times$ 256 $\times$ 2, or nearly an hour and a half.

Now consider how much the process could be speeded up if we filled several rows of k-space during each TR interval. In practice what is, of course, much faster, like going up stairs three steps at a time. Instead of applying the 90 degree pulse for only one row of information in k-space, the 180 degree pulse is applied many times after each 90 degree pulse along with a varying Y gradient before each echo. This way, multiple lines of k-space can be filled during each TR interval. The number of times the 180 degree pulse is applied in each TR interval is called the *echo train length* (ETL). For the FLAIR scan that took over an hour, using an ETL of 10 would reduce the total scan time to less than 9 minutes.

While many imagers were reluctant to say goodbye to their familiar conventional T2 spin echo images, the speed advantage of FSE T2 was just too great to pass up. In addition, some sequences, such as FLAIR, would not be practical without FSE because they require a very long TR time. With conventional spin echo imaging, however, it was quite easy to understand the degree of T2 weighting for each sequence since it was largely based on the time to echo (TE) value. If the TE was long, say more than 50 msec, and the TR was also long, the scan was considered a T2 weighted scan. If the TE interval was short and the TR was long, the pulse sequence was called *proton density weighted*. While that name suggested that it was only capable of depicting the water distribution, remember that all sequences have several factors contributing to contrast, and because a TR time of 2000 msec or so was not particularly long for cerebrospinal fluid (CSF), this sequence was particularly useful for characterization of long T2 lesions.

Predicting the T2 weighting of an image using FSE T2 techniques now becomes much more difficult since a whole series of 180 pulses occur after each 90 degree pulse. Which of the many 180 degree pulses will determine how the image will appear? Since we control all the "instruments" in our MR jazz band, the degree of T2 weighting can be determined by how we link the number of the echo in the echo train with the magnitude of the phase gradient. For example, if we choose to apply a small phase gradient (that will fill a line in the center of k-space) with an early 180 degree pulse, then the scan will appear to be proton density weighted. That is because the small TE echoes will provide only mild *effective* T2 weighting, and it is the center of k-space that determines image contrast. This, of course, means that the stronger phase gradients (that will be assigned to the bottom and top of k-space, which provide detail) are applied with the later echoes. These echoes have a low signal-to-noise ratio precisely because they are long TE echoes, where one expects to recover less signal. This arrangement of using the low signal-to-noise echoes for detail and the high signal-to -noise echoes for image contrast is exactly wrong, so the image quality of FSE proton density MR scans was predictably poor. The T2-weighted FSE technique, on the other hand, reverses the assignment of the small and large phase shifts. By using the first few echoes where there is a lot of signal for the top and bottom of k-space (detail) and the later echoes to fill the center of k-space (contrast), it takes advantage of the best of both. This explains why FSE T2 imaging looks so good. It also reminds me of my father's saying: "Heaven has a Swiss train line and an Italian chef; hell has an Italian train line and a Swiss chef"––although I do have fond memories of many fine dinners I enjoyed with my dear Swiss friends, so I offer it only to make a point.

K-space does not necessarily need to be filled line by line. Just as there is more than one way to mow a lawn or eat corn on the cob, several current techniques fill the center portion of k-space first and in creative ways. This approach has some real advantages for MRA sequences where fast acquisition is critical and contrast trumps detail. In fact, some fast imaging sequences use only partial filling of k-space. Remember that k-space is not a topographic representation of the image. Therefore, if the lower half of k-space is not filled, this does not mean that the lower half of the final image will be blank; it just means that less information will be available.

Another elegant use of k-space that uses partial filling of this space and exploits some advantages of the contrast and detail information involves the motion-correcting sequence called Propeller. By scanning with only partial filling of k-space in a fashion much like the blades of a propeller so that a portion of the center of k-space is included with each sampling, each separate measurement can be registered with the others. This has proven to be very effective for correcting specific types of motion (Figures 1.18 and 1.19).

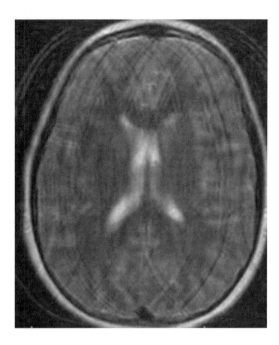

Figure 1.18

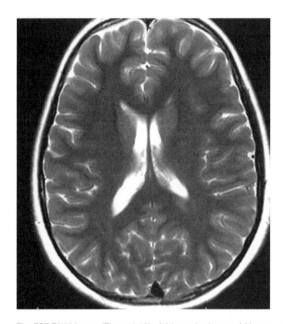

Figure 1.19

The FSE T2WI image (Figure 1.18) of this awake 4-year-old boy was significantly degraded by motion. The patient moved just as much during his propeller T2WI (Figure 1.19) obtained a few minutes later, but using the motion correction capabilities of that particular pulse sequence provided a much better quality image without visible blurring.

Gradient Echo Pulse Sequences

Up to this point, we have relied, just as all early MR scanners did, on the 180 degree pulse to create a spin echo in order to maximize the collection of signal at the antenna. Spin echo sequences, however, because of their 180 degree pulse and subsequent wait for the echo, limit the speed of scan acquisition by requiring a minimum TR time. As magnet homogeneity improved with the widespread use of superconducting magnets, however, it became possible to do away with the 180 degree pulse and create images using only a *gradient echo* instead of the spin echo. It turns out that just by reversing the X gradient, for example, and dropping the 180 degree pulse altogether, an effective echo can be detected at the antenna. The use of gradient echoes allowed the use of shorter TR and TE times and, as a consequence, a significant decrease in scan time. While there are drawbacks to this technique, including increased susceptibility artifacts, the opportunities it created justified the trade-offs.

Apart from saving time, gradient echo imaging presents new possibilities to create contrast. Since the TR times can now be 10 times shorter, a brief application of the RF can still provide enough signal for imaging. This *partial flip angle imaging* has proven to be an important imaging variable.

How can we can recover signal with partial flip angle techniques since we have established that only those spins in the transverse plane relative to the strong magnetic field can induce current in the antenna? This can happen because when we say that the scan was acquired with a 45 degree RF pulse, which seems like the hydrogen protons were tipped only halfway to the transverse plane, we are really talking about the net displacement of a large number of spins. Remember the confusion that may occur if you mix the notion of a single spin with the net magnetization of a great many hydrogen spins. You could think of a 45 degree pulse as roughly equivalent to energizing only half of the potential spins into the 90 degree plane while the other half stayed in their resting state. A more familiar scenario would be to describe a large family as *half way* to Grandma's house when half of them are still at home packing and the other half are sipping hot chocolate by the fire with Grandma.

The option of using less than a 90 degree flip angle (FA) represents another variable that can be modified to influence image contrast. The very short TR times enabled by the use of a small FA and with a short TE, however, means that there may still be some spins in the 90 degree plane from an earlier RF pulse at the time the following RF pulse arrives. These residual spins in the transverse plane will contribute to overall signal, so they need to be considered when a gradient pulse sequence is constructed to highlight specific types of contrast.

With regard to image contrast, a particular gradient echo imaging technique may or may not take advantage of the leftover protons that remain in the transverse plane between RF pulses. We can compare gradient echo imaging to a juggler who, to provide the dramatic touch, has chosen flaming torches. When performing gradient echo imaging, if the residual magnetization is unwelcome, a spoiler pulse is used between applications of the RF pulses to eliminate the residual magnetization. This is how T1-weighted sequences like fast low angle shot (FLASH) or spoiled gradient recalled (SPGR) are acquired. This spoiler effect would be much like knocking the torches out of the air each time the juggler gets three in the air and forcing him to start all over again.

On the other hand, for some applications, this residual magnetization is desirable. In that case, the repeated RF pulses can be used to provide additional energy to offset the natural decay of signal in what is called *steady-state free precession*. This can be exaggerated by correcting all phase shifts to create very strong T2 weighting for sequences like fast imaging employing steady-state acquisition (FIESTA). To continue with the juggler analogy, steady-state imaging would be as if every time the juggler drops a torch or one goes out, an assistant throws him a new lit one so that the number of torches in the air always stays the same, but with a with a mix of old and new torches.

Image Contrast

At this point, we are ready to make images of the body. We have moved beyond the recovery of a simple waveform from the magnetic nuclei in a sample to being able to identify the precise location of that signal. But if all we do is to map the distribution of water in a body, remarkable as that might be, MR would have much less to offer for medical diagnosis. For clinical imaging, we need both detail and contrast between normal tissue and abnormal tissue. In fact, contrast is usually much more important that detail (consider the power of nuclear medicine imaging). If one could design an imaging tool where everything normal on the image was black and everything that was not appeared white, there would be much less need for a lot of detail. In practice, the identification of abnormalities on MR is based on a mix of both alterations of normal structure and signal intensity.

Magnetic resonance scanners can provide contrast using at least seven sources of contrast. These are T1 and T2 relaxation times, proton density, flow, magnetic susceptibility, diffusion, chemical shift, and magnetization transfer. Keep in mind that all MR images combine elements of all of these sources but are designed to exaggerate one or two. For example, diffusion-weighted images are designed to depict the degree of movement of the hydrogen nuclei, but there always remains some element of T2 and susceptibility weighting, particularly if an echo planar technique is used for the acquisition. This is why pulse sequences are described as *weighted*, as in *T1-weighted imaging* (T1WI).

It is essential that the imager be aware of the complexity and richness of MR images in order to avoid making conclusions based on the appearance of a lesion on one or even two of the pulse sequences. If only the T2WI image of the brain were available, for example, it would be very difficult to distinguish an aneurysm (low signal from intravoxel dephasing) from an old hemorrhage (low signal from the susceptibility effect of hemosiderin) or air (low proton density). Let's review the nature of simple T1 and T2 contrast on MR images to establish some basic principles of contrast weighting.

Rotating Frame of Reference

In order to describe more easily how the gradients and RF transmitter in the scanner are used to create contrast, we need some way to illustrate the interaction of the scanner with the hydrogen spins.

(a)

(b)

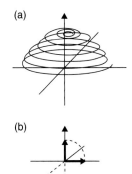

Figure 1.20 At rest, the net magnetic force of the hydrogen nuclei point straight up in this illustration as they align with the strong magnetic field of the MR scanner. A resonant 90 degree pulse, however, would add energy to their pre-existing motion (called precession) which alters their direction of rotation into the perpendicular plane (a). This effect is difficult to illustrate and the depiction of this change can be greatly simplified using a drawing that presumes that the viewer is spinning at the same frequency as the hydrogen called a "rotating frame of reference" (b).

The pulse sequence diagrams tell us what is going on in the scanner hardware but not much about its effect on the hydrogen nuclei. This can be challenging to illustrate because of the complex motions of these spinning objects. Think of how difficult it would be to draw the exact movements in space of a child's waving hand while the child is sitting on a wooden horse going around as well as up and down on a merry-go-round while you are sitting on a nearby park bench. Obviously, this task would be simplified enormously if you could draw that movement while sitting on a bench attached to the platform of the merry-go-round. So, let's simplify this drawing of the motion of the hydrogen nuclei by drawing them while we are hypothetically seated on a bench spinning at precisely the same frequency as the hydrogen nuclei. By using this *rotating frame of reference*, it is relatively easy to depict the effects of the RF pulses on the hydrogen spins that are used to create image contrast (Figure 1.20).

T1 and T2 Relaxation Times

T1 relaxation time, or *spin-lattice relaxation time*, is a fundamental characteristic of tissue, like color or mass. Be careful not to confuse this with TR time, which is the interval between the RF pulses. The T1 time is the time necessary for about two-thirds of the hydrogen spins to return to baseline after being energized with the RF pulse. By the time twice the T1 relaxation time has elapsed, about 90% of the spins have recovered to baseline. At three times the T1 relaxation time, almost all the spins are back where they started. Remember that fluids like CSF have the longest T1 relaxation time encountered in clinical imaging, while fat has one of the shortest. T1 relaxation times are relatively consistent on any scanner but are not absolute, however, since they are influenced by the field strength. This accounts in part for the difficulties of creating MR images with good T1 contrast at 3.0 T compared with imaging at 1.5 T or 0.15 T, for that matter.

T2 relaxation time is another property of tissue and is often called *spin-spin relaxation time*. T2 is the time it takes for two-thirds of the hydrogen nuclei to lose their phase coherence. Remember that just after the 90 degree pulse is turned off, all the energized spins are pointing in the same direction in the state of phase coherence. Because of their degree of order, the signal of the energized hydrogen nuclei will combine to create a strong (well, for a group of tiny atomic nuclei) magnetic field. But with all ordered systems, like a clothes closet or a marching band, without constant reordering this ordered state will unravel. The T2 time is distinct from the T1 time since the hydrogen spins can lose phase coherence while remaining a higher energy state. The two properties are related, however, in the sense that the T2 relaxation time can never be longer than the T1 relaxation time since phase is insignificant once the hydrogen nuclei have returned to their baseline state.

Along with the loss of phase coherence comes a drop in the composite net magnetic field from the energized protons and therefore a decrease in the amplitude of the signal detected in the antenna. Two things account for the rate at which phase coherence is lost. One is the exchange of energy between nearby nuclei (*spin-spin interaction*). This is the reason that the T2 value for water is longer than that for, say, muscle. It reflects the fact that muscle, unlike water, is a highly structured tissue and therefore many of the hydrogen nuclei are in close proximity, facilitating their exchange of energy. The second important factor is the slight but significant irregularity in the homogeneity of the large external magnetic field. This is really a combination of the imperfections in the magnet with distortions caused by the various tissues in the human body. Wherever the field is slightly higher or lower than the native field strength, the protons there will speed ahead or lag behind, depending on the exact magnetic field at their location. This, of course, will also make them go out of phase. These two factors, spin-spin interactions and irregularities in the magnetic field, contribute to dephasing and together are called *T2* relaxation*, which is always shorter than T2 relaxation.

You can think of *T1 relaxation* as somewhat analogous to the time it might take to spend the first $61 of a $100 ATM withdrawal. That time depends in no small way on your location (lattice); i.e., the return to baseline (no cash) would be faster in New York City than in most other places. And once it is gone, there is no getting it back. T2* relaxation can be thought of as a redistribution of the money. It's like giving it to close family members. It is still around, just not in your pocket, and there is a good chance that some of it could be recovered if necessary.

The signal loss due to T2* relaxation can be recovered in part using a *spin echo* pulse sequence. By utilizing a 180 degree pulse, the hydrogen nuclei can be directed to reverse the direction of their rotation. Assuming that the hydrogen spins don't move, and since wherever the magnetic field is strong they will spin back faster and wherever it is weak they will spin back more slowly, this reversal will result in a spin echo (Figure 1.21).

This same principle can be used for a bike ride that includes riders of different abilities who all want to meet for coffee at the end. If everyone starts at the coffee shop and rides at his or her desired or achievable pace, the group of riders will soon spread out, with the fastest at the front of the pack. However, if at the beginning every rider had been instructed to turn around on a signal sent to his or her cell phone and head directly back to the start, using the same route and pace, they would all arrive simultaneously at the coffee shop. That is because even though the faster riders have gone farther than the slow riders, the fast riders will also go back fast, the slow riders go back slow, and everyone should arrive at the start together.

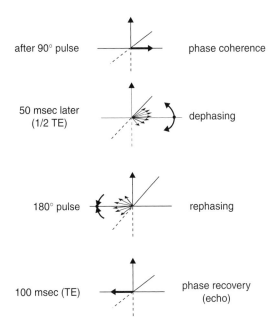

after 90° pulse — phase coherence

50 msec later (1/2 TE) — dephasing

180° pulse — rephasing

100 msec (TE) — phase recovery (echo)

Figure 1.21 The image at the top has an arrow which represents the net magnetization of the hydrogen nuclei immediately after a 90 degrees pulse when they are in coherent phase. In the next frame down, the spins begin to lose their phase coherence and fan out but note how they are still in the transverse plane. After the 180 degree pulse (third from top) which acts like the signal to the riders to return for coffee, the spins will reverse direction so that they converge to form a single net magnetization vector (bottom image) that is detected somewhat later the antenna. Because of this time lag it is called a spin echo.

T1-Weighted Imaging

So, even though we can only examine hydrogen nuclei, it turns out that considerable contrast can be demonstrated due to the differences in tissues' T1 and T2 relaxation times. These differences exist because hydrogen nuclei behave differently, depending on how they are bound to other atoms. For example, the hydrogen spins bound in fat have short T1 relaxation times, while those bound in water molecules have quite long T1 times.

If we are to understand how MR imaging can depict those differences in tissue T1 relaxation times, we need to think now in terms of *pulse sequences*. To illustrate how a series of RF signals can provide T1 contrast, we can focus on brain and CSF. While they are close in terms of their overall proton density, or available hydrogen spins, their T1 relaxation times differ by about 10-fold. Cerebrospinal fluid, which is basically water, has a T1 relaxation time of around 3000 msec, while brain T1 relaxation time is closer to 300 msec. After a single 90 degree RF pulse and using a TE of

20 msec, the returning signal from CSF and brain would be quite similar in amplitude and therefore would provide little visible contrast. But if we repeat that 90 degree pulse 600 msec after the first pulse, we would find that very little signal returns from CSF but a strong signal is recovered from brain. This is because, at 600 msec, 90% of the hydrogen spins in the brain would have returned to baseline (since we are at two times its T1 relaxation time; see Figure 1.22). In CSF, at 600 msec, only a small fraction of the hydrogen nuclei have recovered since that time is only one-fifth of its T1 relaxation time. As a result, the CSF appears black and the brain appears gray on T1WI. If you look at a T1-weighted image (Figure 1.23), you will also notice that fat appears even brighter than brain. That is because fat has an even shorter T1 relaxation time than brain. As a result, all of the protons in fat would have recovered when the second RF pulse arrives, which means that more protons are available to create signal than in brain or CSF.

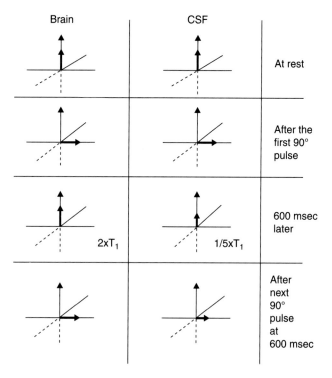

Figure 1.22 The illustration at the top (a) indicates that at rest, brain and CSF have a similar number of available hydrogen spins. After one 90 degree pulse (b) the magnitude of the net magnetization vector for both is therefore similar. Six hundred milliseconds later, brain has effectively recovered, while only a small fraction of the hydrogen spins in CSF have recovered. By initiating a second 90 degree pulse at this point, a relatively large net magnetization vector will be recovered from brain but so few hydrogen spins are now available in CSF that they provide only a small signal at the antenna. This is the reason CSF appears dark (low signal) compared with brain (higher signal) on short TR short TE (T1WI) images.

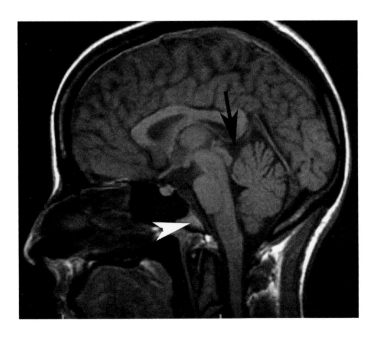

Figure 1.23 This sagittal T1WI shows the expected dark CSF in the subarachnoid spaces (arrow) and ventricles, while the brain provides more signal and is therefore displayed as gray. Note that the marrow fat (arrowhead), because it has an even shorter T1 relaxation time than brain, appears white since all those protons would have recovered completely between the closely spaced 90 degree pulses.

T2 Image Contrast

T2-weighted imaging uses a similar approach for creating contrast from differential recovery but now, of course, based on T2 relaxation times. In order to create images with predominately T2 weighting, we must first minimize the influence of T1 relaxation. For T1 contrast, we used a short TR of 600 msec to make tissue with a long T1 relaxation time appear dark. If we choose a much longer TR time that allows nearly complete recovery of both brain and CSF hydrogen spins, however, we will see very little contrast as long as proton density remains the same. For example, at a TR time of 6000 msec, we will find that there is complete recovery for brain protons and nearly complete recovery for CSF protons. That slight difference occurs because CSF has a T1 relaxation time of 3000 msec, so at a TR of 6000 msec, 90% of the protons there would be available for the next RF pulse. We could, of course, use even longer times, but that comes at the expense of longer scan times.

Now that we have minimized T1 effects, let's consider how to create T2 contrast between brain and CSF. For this discussion, let's say that CSF has a T2 relaxation time of 2000 msec and brain has a T2 relaxation time of 100 msec. To accentuate T2 contrast, we can take advantage of the time delay between the 90 degree pulse and the TE. To create this echo, we will use a 180 degree RF pulse to rephase the spins, remembering that the TE time is twice the interval between the 90 and 180 degree pulses.

For protons in brain, with a T2 time of 100 msec, there would be very little phase coherence left to recover if we listen for signal after 200 msec. This is because at that point in time, i.e., twice the T2 for brain, 90% of the hydrogen spins would have lost their phase coherence (Figure 1.24). If we go back to the cycling analogy, so much time would have gone by when the turnaround signal arrived that most of the riders would have already loaded their bikes in their cars, and some would already be driving home. At the same TE of 200 msec, however, only a small proportion the CSF protons (TE of 2000 msec) would have lost their phase coherence, so the 180 degree RF pulse would create a strong echo. This strong returning signal from the CSF will be represented with bright pixels on the T2 weighted scan, while the brain will appear dark.

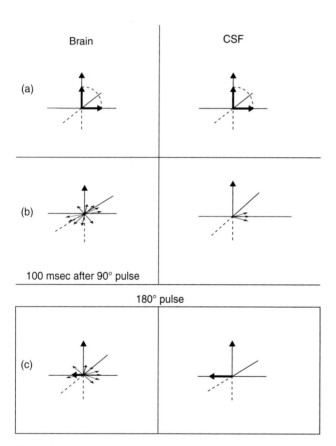

Figure 1.24 This illustration compares how the T2 relaxation times of brain and CSF behave on a T2WI. In the upper row note that the net magnetization of spins in brain and CSF after a 90 degree pulse appear similar, i.e. both are in the transverse plane and all spins point in the same direction (phase coherent). In the second row, 100 msec later, the phase of those spins in brain, while still in the transverse plane, have dispersed, resulting in considerable loss of signal since the spins will now cancel each other out. This would provide in very small net magnetization (signal) at the antenna. Loss of phase coherence of this magnitude cannot be recovered with a 180 degree pulse. On your right in that row, however, notice how little dephasing has occurred in CSF. This is because CSF has a very long T2 relaxation time. This small drift in phase, after a rephasing 180 degree pulse (see bottom row), will provide a strong echo and therefore signal at the antenna which accounts for the high signal of CSF on T2WI.

Inversion Recovery

Inversion recovery (IR) is another basic MR imaging technique that is used to bring out different patterns of contrast. It uses an additional 180 degree pulse that occurs before the 90 degree pulse. The two IR sequences that are most common in clinical use are STIR (short tau inversion recovery) and FLAIR (fluid-attenuated inversion recovery) imaging. The time interval between the initial 180 degree pulse and the 90 degree pulse is called the *time to inversion* (TI). These are both spin echo sequences, so there is a 180 degree pulse that occurs before and after the 90 degree pulse.

A 180 degree pulse can be created by doubling the intensity or duration of the 90 degree RF pulse. When in the 180 degree orientation, the spins will provide no signal because only spins in the transverse plane can create current in the antenna. This may seem counterintuitive since twice as much energy is absorbed by the protons. You should also keep in mind that as the spins recover and return to their resting state, they still will not provide signal until we apply a 90 degree pulse.

Now, consider what might happen if that 90 degree pulse occurs precisely when net magnetization for CSF is moving through the zero point in its recovery path (Figure 1.25). Since at this point there would be no available hydrogen spins to move into the transverse plane, CSF will appear dark. This is the basis for FLAIR imaging, where normal CSF signal is suppressed, although the image is otherwise T2 weighted. If we choose a short TI time so that the 90 degree pulse occurs when hydrogen spins in fat are at their zero point in recovery, we will now have a STIR scan with dark fat.

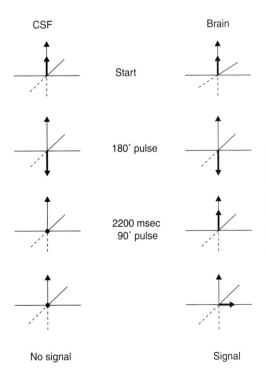

Figure 1.25 At the start (top row) both CSF and brain have similar net magnetization at rest. After the 180 degree pulse (second row from top), their magnetic vectors now point down, so no signal is recovered at the antenna since no spins are moving in the transverse plane. To generate current in the antenna, a 90 degree pulse will be necessary. If this occurs 2200 msec after the 180 degree pulse (third row), the net magnetization for those spins in CSF is zero based on their predictable T1 relaxation time. Since no spins are available, no signal will be provided by CSF spins after the 90 degree pulse (bottom row). Compare this with brain. At the same TI of 2200 msec, brain is well along with longitudinal recovery (right image, third row), so a larger number of spins are available for imaging. After the 90 degree pulse, brain will therefore provide signal and appears gray, while CSF is black on a FLAIR scan. After the 90 degree pulse a second 180 degree pulse is used to recover signal for this spin echo sequence.

Magnet Safety

METAL

One of the critical responsibilities of all MR staff and technologists is ensuring magnet safety since the powerful magnetic fields used for imaging present a serious risk to patients and staff. The three pillars of MR safety are training all personnel who might come into the MR suite, limiting access to the scanner suite, and maintaining constant vigilance. Each institution has its own guidelines for access and patient screening; they should be carefully considered in order to minimize the risk to both patients and staff.

The danger associated with MR scanners is magnified because their strong magnetic field is unlike anything else in our daily experience and because the field is completely invisible. The field strength of an MR magnet is sufficient to pull a pen out of your pocket or lift an oxygen cylinder off the floor (Figure 1.26) and draw them into the scanner bore. This is called the *missile effect*. The risks of this interaction are compounded by the fact that the magnetic field will not only accelerate the movement of the metal object toward the scanner (think of *Star Trek*'s tractor beams) but will also pull it directly into the center of the bore, where there may be a patient.[12]

Of course, not all metal will be attracted. Aluminum is used for MR-compatible oxygen tanks and intravenous (IV) poles since it has no ferromagnetic properties. Unfortunately, aluminum and polished steel may look sufficiently similar that training and awareness are required to recognize the different types of metal, and there is no margin for error.

One very important but routine task that is essential for MR safety is the careful screening of all patients for implanted devices or metal prior to scanning. The goal is to be strict enough so that patients who are truly at risk are excluded but flexible enough so that MR imaging is not denied to those patients who might benefit. This is not simple in practice, and it requires good judgment and some knowledge of metallurgy and medical device technology (YouTube[13] video "Metals and MR Safety MRphysics"). Such decisions must sometimes take into account where the metal is located, the kind of metal, how long it has been there, and the magnitude of the risk to the patient versus the potential benefit. This process becomes particularly difficult when the exact nature of the metal or device cannot be established with certainty prior to the scan.

Consider, for example, a patient with known shotgun pellets in his body (Figures 1.27 and 1.28). While there is obviously radiographic evidence of retained metal, the nature of this metal will determine the risk of an MR scan for this patient. One approach might be to first find out if the patient was shot while hunting ducks or was a victim of urban violence. If the patient was shot while hunting ducks, the odds are that the metal represents a significant risk to the patient having an MR scan. The

12 In my training many years ago, I found gradate students playing "magneto-darts" at lunchtime using their small research magnet. After a piece of thick plywood with standard target scoring rings was placed over the bore of the magnet, a dart could be thrown merely in the direction of the magnet, and it was fascinating to watch even poorly thrown darts pulled directly into the center of the target. (Do not try this at your site; today, no one will be amused.)

13 YouTube video "Metals and MR Safety": http://www.youtube.com/watch?v=Z9bki8zidvw.

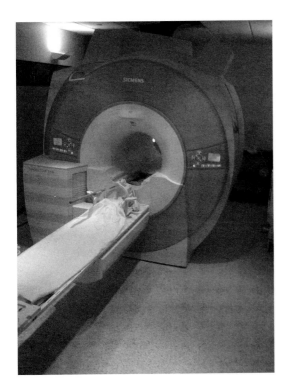

Figure 1.26 This mop, stuck inside the bore, was brought too close to the magnet and it proved to be difficult to pull it out. In the radiology department, it is essential to remember that both X-ray radiation and strong magnetic fields are invisible but ever- present risks to you, your colleagues, and your patients. Unlike similar-sized X-ray devices in the department like CT scanners and angiography units, the strong magnetic field of an MR scanner is never turned off.

reason is that while most shotgun shells are loaded with lead shot, waterfowl hunters cannot use lead shot for environmental reasons and usually use steel shot. This particular patient was shot during a robbery, and since cartridges with steel shot are considerably more expensive and less common than shotgun shells with lead shot, this patient probably harbors lead shot that has no significant magnetic properties.

Nearly all orthopedic hardware should be safe to scan because it is not only made of nonferrous metal but is also rigidly attached to the skeleton. Titanium is completely safe. The nickel used in stainless steel alloys to keep the steel from rusting also degrades its ferromagnetic properties. (Don't believe it? Try putting a refrigerator magnet on the door of a stainless steel model.) There had been some concern because in vitro testing of large items of surgical hardware has shown that these items will heat up slightly with MR imaging. In vivo this effect is negligible because the circulation of blood should allow this added heat to be conducted away.

With any decision regarding implanted hardware, however, it is essential to listen to the patient. Pay careful attention to any patient who reports a sensation of heat or pain near metal during the course of an MR scan. While you may be right in believing that a specific implant or metal is safe, you will eventually encounter circumstances in which the patient experiences symptoms nevertheless, and these should be taken seriously to avoid injury from local heating.

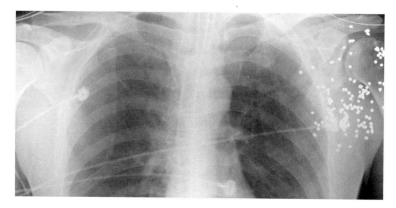

Figure 1.27

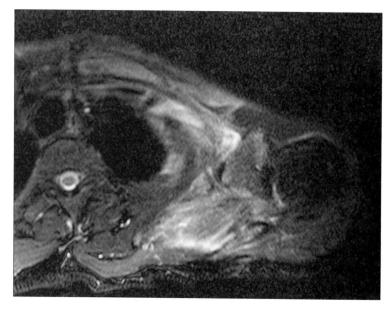

Figure 1.28

While this patient had been shot in the shoulder (Figure 1.27) his MR scan (Figure 1.28) was uneventful because this was lead shot with no magnetic properties.

While orthopedic hardware is firmly attached to the skeleton, metal in soft parts of the body like the eye and brain may present a serious risk to the patient. There are rare reports of blindness and death from movement of retained metal in the eye and a cerebral aneurysm clip that proved to be ferromagnetic. While all current production aneurysm clips approved for use in the United States must meet specific requirements that ensure their safety for routine clinical MR scanning, it is prudent and standard practice to identify the type of clip that each patient harbors. This becomes particularly important if the patient had surgery at another institution or in past decades. Be careful in obtaining this history since the patient may have had more than one surgery with placement of multiple clips. Unlike aneurysm clips, the coils used for endovascular treatment of aneurysms are not only safe to scan, but MR is the preferred study for imaging follow-up at many centers. These detachable coils are made of platinum, a metal that, like titanium, is also completely safe in the MR environment since it has no ferromagnetic properties.

Currently, there is a large and growing number of implanted electrical devices to contend with as well. These include deep brain stimulators, adjustable ventriculoperitoneal (VP) shunts, pacemakers, intraspinal pumps, and vagal nerve stimulators. It is important to ask the patient open-ended questions to determine whether he or she has an implanted device and, if so, exactly what type. It is not sufficient, for example, to determine that a patient has VP shunt. Many newer VP shunts are adjustable, and since the valve settings are changed using a magnet, these devices may need to be reset after the patient's MR scan. An excellent resource in making these decisions is the Web site http://www.MRIsafety.com, but you should also learn to use the manufacturer's Web site and published literature to determine whether there is significant risk to the patient or the integrity of the device. This analysis should also include such factors as whether a send and receive coil is used, what body part is imaged, and the scanner power deposition necessary to make the diagnosis. For example, while cardiac pacemakers were once considered an absolute contraindication for MR scanning, some sites now offer MR scanning to a select group of patients, with specific pacemakers, using strictly defined guidelines and scanner techniques.

MISSILE EFFECT

Metal in the scanner room can also represent a risk to the patient or technologist if it is ferromagnetic and mistakenly brought near the MR scanner. Patients should be advised to leave behind all accessories of modern life like cell phones, watches, pens, and the like. Taking a fine old gold watch or credit cards into the scanner does not necessarily pose a risk to the patient, but when the watch stops or the credit card data are erased, no one will be happy. Requiring all patients to change into a gown, even when not necessarily essential for the scan, may be helpful to avoid such accidents. It may not be immediately obvious, but if even small items like bobby pins or paper clips end up inside the scanner cowling, you may encounter puzzling image quality problems until they are found.

Much more dangerous are accidents in which large metal objects are drawn rapidly into the scanner. There are a variety of scenarios in which this can occur, and it is much more common than one would appreciate from the literature. This is because the vast majority of these accidents that occur without injury go unreported. Over the course of my career, I have seen or heard of quite a few, and I am aware of many more near calamities that were averted by clear-thinking MR technologists. The most serious as well as among the most common ones involve oxygen tanks.

Medical oxygen tanks (Figure 1.29) are ubiquitous in both hospital and outpatient settings. One reason they present such problems is that the steel and aluminum tanks are sufficiently similar in appearance to be confused in an emergency.

Even the decision of some hospital administrators to stock only nonferrous tanks may create another problem since the MR staff may then believe that all the oxygen tanks they encounter are MR compatible. However, ambulance and helicopter transport will inevitably bring into the hospital environment ferrous oxygen of tanks from outside, so careful evaluation of every tank that comes near the MR suite is essential. The greatest risk seems to occur when a well-meaning individual mistakenly brings the closest oxygen tank he or she can find into the scanner room for a patient in distress. One reported death has been attributed to this situation, and it is likely that many other near accidents have been averted. This is another reason why any patient in distress should be quickly moved outside the scanner.

The technologists provide the last and best screening of all staff who enter the MR room. It is important to empower them to challenge anyone who walks into the scanner room, without regard to their manner or rank, if they have not been cleared. This problem is not limited to medical personnel. There have been reports of rescue and housekeeping personnel, as well as police, bringing

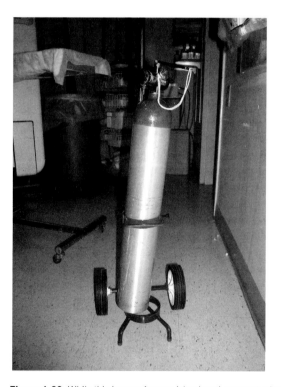

Figure 1.29 While this is a nonferrous (aluminum) oxygen tank and can therefore enter the MR scanner room, be aware that it may be sitting in a ferrous cart.

a variety of hardware into the scanner room, sometimes with subsequent injury. Adequate control of room access, an understanding of why some metals are safe and others are dangerous, and how to tell the difference are critical responsibilities of the MR staff that should avert these sometimes comical, often dangerous, and nearly always expensive accidents.

RF BURNS

Less commonly encountered but potentially quite serious are patient burns that can occur during MR scanning due to power deposition. Body heating is generally not an issue in healthy adults, but significant heating may occur when imaging children or when wires are directly on the patient's skin surface. There are reports of many such burns on the FDA Web site[14] associated with electrocardiogram wires and pulse oximeters. It is essential that any wires near the patient be isolated from the skin surface by blankets or towels. In addition, wires in the scanner should be straightened to avoid formation of loops, which increases RF heating effects.

POWER OFF VERSUS QUENCH

Rarely, usually during the process of filling with liquid helium, if just one small region of the wire wrap loses its property of superconduction, it will suddenly get hot due to the normal heating from electrical resistance. As this section of wire warms, that heat will make the adjacent wire wraps warm up. This widening zone of warming can quickly heat the whole magnet, resulting in sudden boiling off of the liquid helium and loss of superconduction. The conversion of a large volume of liquid helium into a much larger volume of helium gas with loss of superconduction is called a *quench* (Figures 1.30 and 1.31). This slow-motion explosion is associated with an unforgettable roaring sound as the helium gas is (hopefully) diverted outside the scanner room through a specially designed vent pipe. A quench almost never occurs intentionally because this sudden release of energy involves a significant risk of damage to the integrity of the magnet casing and wiring, as well as to anyone who is in the room. This is because there is a risk of suffocation from displacement of oxygen in the room by helium if there is even a small leak or fracture in the vent pipe. There are also the costs to consider, which can be very large if there is permanent damage to the superconducting wire from heat and twisting, as well as the predictable loss of all of the expensive liquid helium in the Dewar.

The risks, not to mention the costs, of a quench make it impractical to be used as a strategy in dealing with a patient in distress. For those of you who work daily with MR scanners, it is essential to recognize the difference between turning the scanner's power off and quenching the magnet. Turning the electrical power off is the correct decision when there is concern about a fire or a short circuit in the scanner. Since the magnet at nearly all sites is superconducting and therefore is not linked to the power supply, this will *not* turn the magnet off. In fact, the only situation in which an emergency quench should be considered is the unlikely circumstance of someone actually pinned in the magnet by a large metal object or a similar extraordinary crisis. As a rule, the patient should be moved out of the scanner whenever there is a medical need that must be quickly addressed.

14 FDA, Medical Devices, MRI: http://www.fda.gov/cdrh/safety/mrisafety.html.

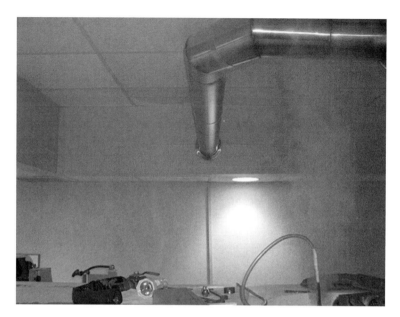

Figure 1.30

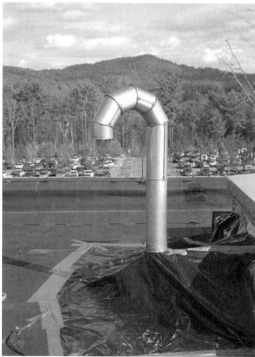

Figure 1.31

Figure 1.30 was taken soon after a 1.5 T magnet quenched during a helium refill. Note the horizontal crack in the wall where the pipe exits the room into the wall. This was caused by the sudden expansion of the pipe as it filled with helium gas during the quench. No one was hurt, and the magnet sustained no lasting damage in this particular event. That same rapid expansion of the vent pipe also dislodged a section of the hospital roof (Figure 1.31). While this took some time to repair, as quenching a magnet goes, these damages were considered minor.

Suggested Readings

Chaljub G, Kramer LA, Johnson RF III, et al. Projectile cylinder accidents resulting from the presence of ferromagnetic nitrous oxide or oxygen tanks in the MR suite. *AJR*. 2001;177:27–30.

Damadian R. Tumor detection by nuclear magnetic resonance. *Science*. 1971;171:1151–1153.

Forbes KP, Pipe JG, Karis JP, et al. Brain imaging in the unsedated pediatric patient: comparison of periodically rotated overlapping parallel lines with enhanced reconstruction and single-shot fast spin-echo sequences. *AJNR*. 2003;24:794–798.

Klucznik RP, Carrier DA, Pyka R, et al. Placement of a ferromagnetic intracerebral aneurysm clip in a magnetic field with a fatal outcome. *Radiology*. 1993;187:855–856.

Mezrich R. A perspective on K-space. *Radiology*. 1995;195:297–315.

Shellock FG, Curtis JS. MR imaging and biomedical implants, materials, and devices: an updated review. *Radiology*. 1991;180:541–550.CT

2 MR ARTIFACTS

In the cases that follow, you will find discussions of MR techniques designed to emphasize contrast due to flow, diffusion, susceptibility, chemical shift, and magnetization transfer contrast. Always keep in mind that MR images contain a wealth of information that will be more accessible to those who examine them with a keen eye and a good understanding of how they were created.

Artifact 1

This 64-year-old woman presents with new symptoms of leg numbness. Her MR scan of the cervical spine was normal with the exception of one section (Figure A1.1) at the bottom of the axial T1WI stack that is depicted on the sagittal scan (Figure A1.2).

You think the high signal in the spinal canal is most likely to represent:

(1) an intradural meningioma.

(2) a flow-related artifact.

(3) an arachnoid cyst.

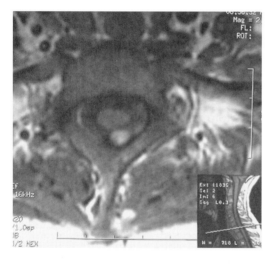

Figure A1.1

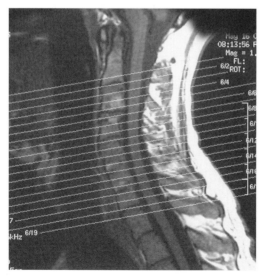

Figure A1.2

FLOW-RELATED ENHANCEMENT

It is important to consider how this particular slice relates to the stack of axial images, particularly when you consider that the other pulse sequences were normal. This finding most likely is due to a CSF flow-related artifact. While you may be familiar with some of the flow effects in blood vessels, there are CSF flow artifacts to contend with as well. Because of these flow effects, you should approach all lesions you see on the first one or two slices on either side of a stack of images with skepticism.

Flow-related enhancement can be explained using the concepts we reviewed to explain T1-related contrast. To create T1-weighted contrast, the interval between the 90 degree pulses needs to be short enough that only tissues with a short T1 relaxation will have enough time to return to their rest state. Their quick recovery time allows nearly all of the hydrogen spins to be ready and available for next RF pulse. In CSF, on the other hand, T1 recovery time is so long that only a small fraction of the total available hydrogen protons will be available for the next 90 degree RF pulse. Keep in mind, however, that this technique for highlighting T1 contrast is based on the assumption that the hydrogen spins are stationary.

If new batches of spins arrive from outside the imaging volume and move into the imaging slice alongside the stationary spins, they can provide much more signal than their stationary neighbors (Figures A1.3 and A1.4). Think of them as fresh players coming off the bench in the second half of a ball game. While the stationary spins in that slice have been beaten up by the repeated 90 degree pulses, nearly all of the spins coming from outside are available for imaging. In the next 90 degree pulse or so, they provide more signal than their tired neighbors, creating *flow-related enhancement* in the entry slice (Figure A1.5). As they course through the imaging volume, however, they will soon behave like their neighbors after they have experienced repeated 90 degree pulses. Entry slice enhancement is important to recognize so that it is not mistaken for an abnormal structure but, at the same time, does not simply represent a nuisance for MR imagers. It can provide information about the direction of flow and the presence of flow, and we will see that it is the basis for contrast on all time- of-flight MRA imaging.

Correct answer: 2

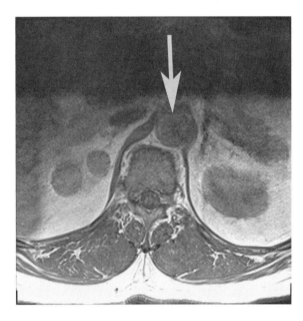

Figure A1.3

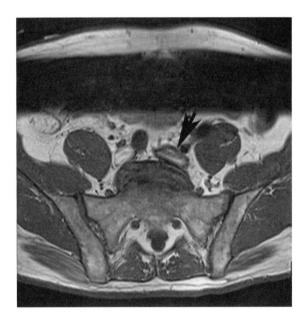

Figure A1.4

Figure A1.3 is the first slice at the top of a stack of axial images of the abdomen; Figure A1.4 is the last slice at the bottom. Note that the aorta (arrow) appears brighter than the inferior vena cava on this top slice (Figure A1.3). This is due to the entry slice effect since the blood in the aorta is flowing into this slice with a full complement of fresh hydrogen spins. At the bottom slice of the stack, the blood in the aorta is now dark, having experienced multiple 90 degree pulses as it traversed the volume, while the signal in the iliac veins (Figure A1.4, arrow) is bright since that blood is just entering the imaging volume from below.

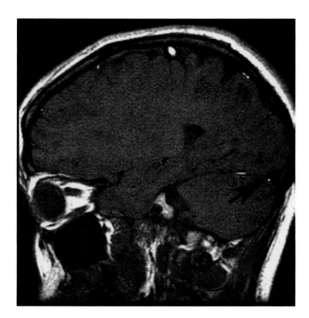

Figure A1.5 Entry slice effects can be helpful to indicate the direction of flow. On this sagittal T1WI image, notice that the cortical veins are all bright due to entry slice enhancement because the direction of flow in these veins runs from lateral to medial going toward the superior sagittal sinus. It is important to recognize, therefore, that the transverse sinus (arrow) should appear black since blood flow there runs in the opposite direction (medial to lateral). High signal in the transverse sinus may indicate either thrombosis or reversed flow due an occlusion of the sigmoid sinus or jugular bulb. In any event, it usually warrants further investigation.

Artifact 2

This 44-year-old male presents with long-standing and progressively worsening bilateral leg weakness. The clinician, who is well known for his diagnostic acumen, orders an MR scan with the indication "rule out spinal dural-arterial fistula." You notice these dark areas in the CSF on both the axial (Figure A2.1) and sagittal (Figure A2.2) T2WI images and attribute this low signal to:

(1) spinal vascular malformation.

(2) blood products in the subarachnoid space.

(3) intravoxel dephasing.

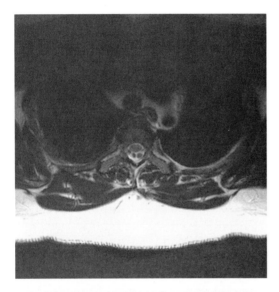

Figure A2.1

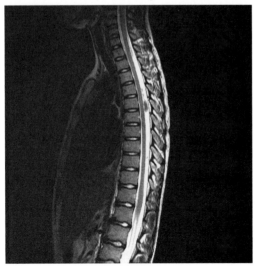

Figure A2.2

This finding of low signal within the CSF in the dorsal thoracic subarachnoid space is very common on T2WI if you care to look for it. Like many findings on imaging, it may get unwarranted attention if you happen to look there for the first time when the history suggests a spinal vascular lesion. We expect the CSF to appear bright on T2WI because of its long T2 relaxation time. By waiting a bit after the 90 degree pulse, we will recover more signal from the CSF than the surrounding tissues because the protons in those tissues with shorter T2 relaxation times will lose their phase coherence more quickly than CSF.

Prior to the use of routine MR imaging, the vigorous pulsation of CSF was not really appreciated by most imagers (Figures A2.3–A2.5). As it moves in distinct flow channels, CSF will appear dark from flow-related loss of phase coherence. You should recall that the gradients are applied repeatedly in order to encode spatial information into the returning signal. While the pulse diagrams in Chapter 1 are simplified, in practice the gradients for slice selection and frequency encoding are applied not once but twice. This is done to reverse unwanted phase shifts that occur whenever a gradient is applied.

This balanced reversal of gradients works well to maximize signal from static spins by correcting phase shifts. If the spins are moving about, however, it is unlikely that the second gradient they experience will balance the first. Think of this technique of balanced gradients as analogous to two long lines of impatient travelers waiting at an airport security gate. Now take one dollar from everyone in line 1 and give one dollar to everyone in line 2. Five minutes later, take a dollar from everyone in line 2 and give a dollar to everyone in line 1. The traveler who stayed in his or her original line would be no richer or poorer than at the start. However, someone who jockeyed back and forth to find the fastest line could easily end up ahead or behind by a few dollars, depending on where he or she was when the dollars were coming and going. If we change this analogy to phase instead of dollars, by changing locations, moving hydrogen spins may lose or accumulate phase compared with their neighbors. If we want to maximize the net magnetic field in a voxel, the phase of every proton spinning in the transverse plane should point in the same direction, a condition called *phase coherence*. Protons spinning in the transverse plane but with opposite phase will cancel out, thus decreasing the net magnetic field and therefore the signal. Random phase in a voxel results in no signal coming from that location and will appear as a *signal void*. The loss of phase coherence due to flow in the dorsal subarachnoid space is the cause of these rounded signal voids that are evident in Figures A2.1 and A2.2.

How can normal CSF flow artifacts be differentiated from the abnormal vascular flow voids of a vascular malformation on MR scans? Abnormal vessels tend to be more sharply defined compared with CSF flow artifacts and nearly always (with rare exceptions) demonstrate some enhancement after administration of contrast (Figures A2.6 and A2.7). This is because the venous outflow of many spinal vascular malformations drains via dilated veins that have relatively slow flow, so they will enhance. Another aid to differentiate venous from CSF flow is that symptomatic spinal vascular malformations are almost always associated with focal prolonged T2 relaxation in the cord due to venous hypertension. Solid masses can be encountered in the dorsal subarachnoid space as well so remember that CSF flow effects are usually not evident on T1WI (Figures A2.8–A2.11).

Correct answer: 3. Intravoxel dephasing from CSF flow.

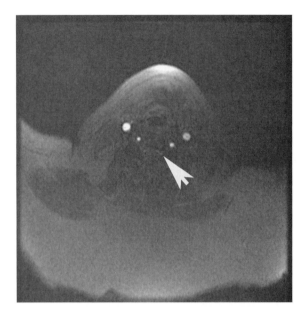

Figure A2.3

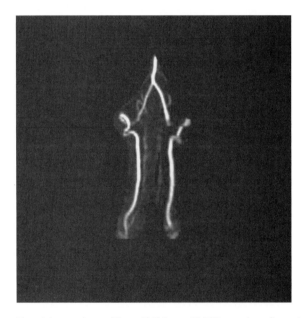

Figure A2.4

The axial source image (Figure A2.3) from a 2D TOF scan shows flow-related enhancement of moving spins within the arteries in the neck. Note that there is also increased signal just anterior to the cord (arrow). When the axial images are reconstructed as a MIP image (Figure A2.4), you can see the vertebral arteries clearly, but notice the parallel bright vertical lines between them. If you consider it for a moment you might find that it looks familiar. That is because it resembles contrast on a cervical myelogram as this signal arises not from vascular flow but from CSF flow around the cord.

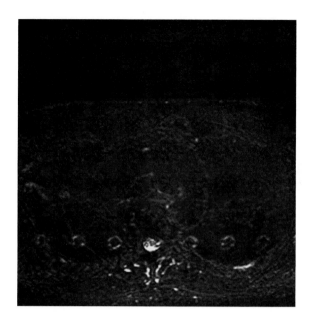

Figure A2.5 This image demonstrates flow-related artifacts arising from CSF pulsations around the cord. Note that the misregistered signal from the CSF projects well away from the canal in the phase direction. This repeating pattern of artifactual structures is called *ghosting*.

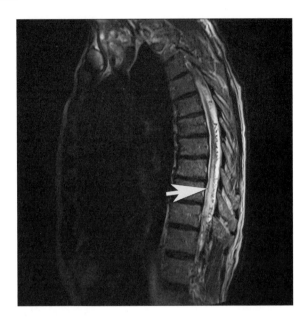

Figure A2.6

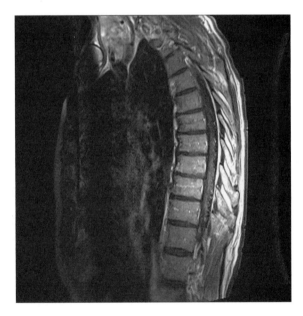

Figure A2.7

The flow voids on the surface of the cord (Figure A2.6) are due to a spinal vascular malformation, not CSF flow. Note that they are sharply defined and small. Also note the abnormal T2 prolongation signal in the cord (arrow). In cases where you suspect a spinal vascular abnormality, ask for a contrast-enhanced scan. On the sagittal T1WI postcontrast scan of the same patient (Figure A2.7), there is dot-like enhancement on the dorsal surface of the cord arising from the large draining vein. This is of considerable significance since CSF flow would never be expected to enhance with an IV contrast agent. Contrast-enhanced spinal MR angiography can be very helpful as well for establishing the diagnosis of a spinal vascular malformation.

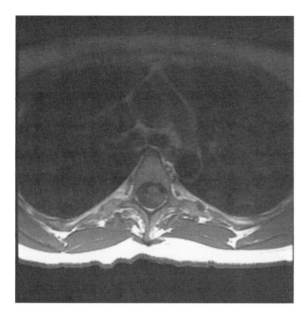

Figure A2.8

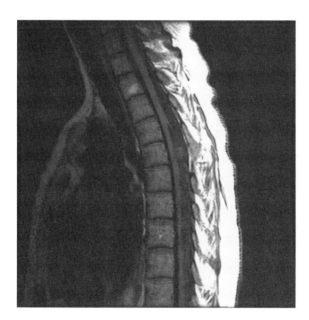

Figure A2.9 This patient also has abnormal signal in the dorsal subarachnoid space. However, these findings should not be mistaken for typical CSF flow artifacts because they should not be this evident on a T1WI. The patient was symptomatic and she went on to have a CT myelogram (Figures A2.10 and A2.11) and then surgery for removal of this neurenteric cyst.

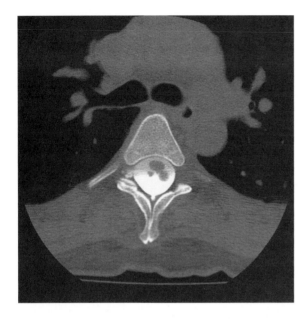

Figure A2.10

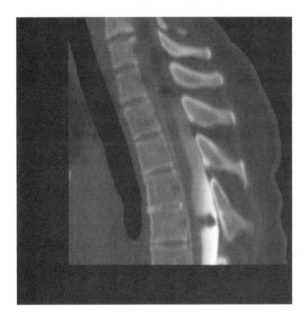

Figure A2.11

Artifact 3

These MR images of patient A (Figure A3.1) and patient B (Figure A3.2) are displayed with the T1-weighted image without contrast on your left and on the right a T1-weighted image with contrast. Select one of the following statements that you believe is true:

(1) Both of these patients have a glomus jugulare tumor.

(2) Neither of these patients has a glomus jugulare tumor.

(3) Patient A has a glomus jugulare tumor, B does not.

(4) Patient B has a glomus jugulare tumor, A does not.

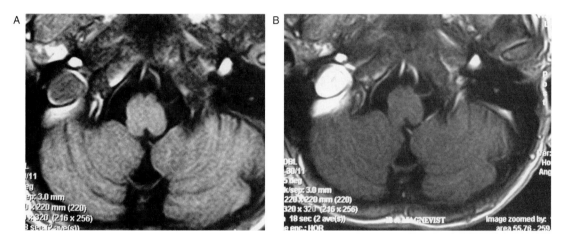

Figure A3.1 Patient A.

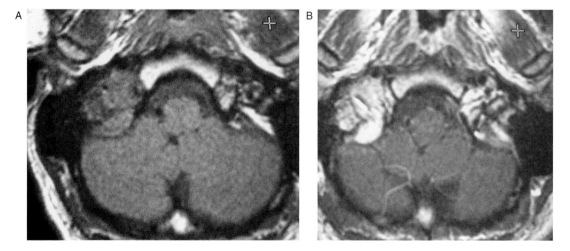

Figure A3.2 Patient B.

IN-PLANE AND SLOW FLOW

We have now seen that flow can appear bright from entry slice effects or dark from intravoxel dephasing. As you might expect, there is a middle situation where blood flow can have intermediate signal and resemble thrombus or tumor. Administration of contrast will not help you in this situation because slowly moving blood will also enhance from the T1 effects of the contrast, as is evident in Figure A3.1.

The jugular bulb is a common site of this artifact, but it is by no means limited to the brain. In this location, however, the asymmetry is due to differences in the velocity of blood flow as well as the anatomic differences in the outflow of the left and right jugular veins.

Intravoxel dephasing, the cause of low signal in fast-moving fluid, is most evident where there is turbulence from high-velocity flow or flow across slices. The intermediate signal in the jugular vein in patient A reflects the fact that the flow in the jugular bulb is both slow and turns a bit within the plane of the section. By staying in the same slice, the protons in blood will experience nearly the same gradients as neighboring spins. I find it helpful to think of slow flow as analogous to a deep pool of water in a fast-flowing brook where you would not expect the surface to have the same ripples on the surface as in the faster flowing shallow portions of the stream.

If you look carefully at the two scans, you will also notice that the tumor in patient B appears inhomogeneous in signal. The low-signal areas reflects small flow voids with intravoxel dephasing due to fast, turbulent flow in the prominent arteries within this highly vascular tumor.

Correct answer: 4

Artifact 4

Figures A4.1 and A4.2 are both T1WI postenhanced sagittal scans and were obtained within minutes of each other, yet the canal and the distal cord are much better seen on Figure A4.1. The difference is due to:

(1) the use of a saturation band.

(2) the use of respiratory gating.

(3) exchange of the phase and frequency encoding directions.

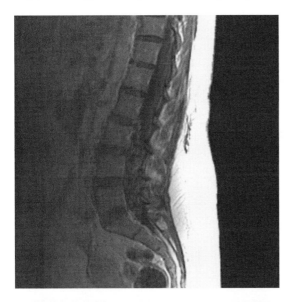

Figure A4.1

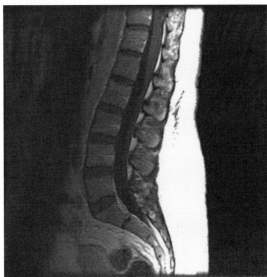

Figure A4.2

PHASE ENCODING

The measure of picture elements (pixels) in each direction of the image is called the *matrix*. If you use very few picture elements (coarse matrix), you may be able to actually see the blocks of information that form the image (Figure A4.3).

Using a matrix with a larger number of picture elements (fine matrix) usually provides a smoother-appearing image in which the individual pixels cannot be easily discriminated.

Magnetic resonance scanners provide choices for image matrix. Since a fine matrix will take more time to acquire but usually involves less signal, the choice of matrix on MR images reflects a compromise among image quality, time, and signal. The pixels do not have to be square, and it is common to use rectangular pixels e.g. matrix choices of 128 x 256 or 256 x 512.

The larger the matrix, the smaller the area of the picture elements if the field of view stays the same. You may have spent some time poring over megapixel numbers if you have been shopping for a high-definition TV or digital camera. As you may have discovered, more pixels usually come with a higher price. But for cameras, TVs and MR scanners, more picture elements do not necessarily mean better pictures. While higher resolution sounds good in principle, for cameras and MR scanners it also means less information available in each pixel. For example, assuming that the lens, light, and subject are the same, dividing the sensor screen of a camera into smaller elements will result in fewer photons arriving in each element. If noise stays constant, then this means that the signal-to-noise ratio may be lower in the latest and greatest camera compared with another camera with a lower megapixel measure. This effect may become particularly apparent in low-light situations.

With MR, smaller picture elements mean that there are fewer hydrogen nuclei per "voxel." This three-dimensional projection of the pixel (voxel) is defined by the face of the pixel and the slice thickness. Decreasing either the slice thickness or the pixel size results in fewer protons per voxel. With fewer hydrogen protons in each voxel, and assuming the noise stays the same, the signal-to-noise ratio decreases, which may decrease image contrast. There are several ways to correct for this loss of signal, however.

The scan time for a simple spin echo acquisition is based on the facts that a 90 degree pulse is necessary for each gradient step and that one gradient step is necessary for each line of information in the phase encoding direction. As a result, a 512 x 512 matrix requires twice as much time to acquire as a 256 x 256 scan but the pixels at 512 x 512 will be one-fourth the size. While it might seem that this would decrease the signal by one-fourth, since each phase encoding step contributes to the signal of the entire image (see discussion of k-space in chapter 1), the signal loss decreases by only one-half since there are twice as many phase encoding steps in a 512 versus a 256 square matrix.

The decrease in the signal-to-noise ratio can be corrected in part by repeating the entire pulse sequence more than once and averaging the results. This variable is sometimes abbreviated as NEX, meaning "number of excitations." Each excitation adds time, of course, so using a NEX of 2 doubles the scan time. You might think that one would double the signal by doubling the scan time. Unfortunately, you still won't come out even because when you double the scan time, the signal-to-noise ratio increases only by a factor of 1.4 (square root of 2), not 2. To double the signal, you would need to use a NEX of 4 or a scan time four times as long (square root of 4 = 2) to break even. For this

Correct answer: 3

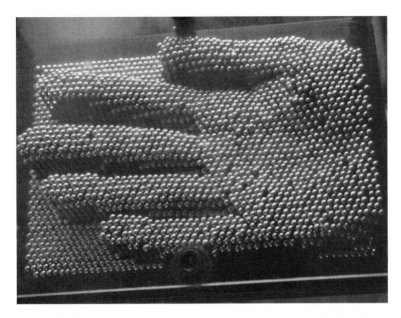

Figure A4.3 This toy made of metal pins is great fun and also demonstrates how the size of the pixels relates to image quality. Had the pins been smaller and more numerous, the curves around the fingers would be represented more accurately and with fewer terraced edges.

reason, it is prudent to avoid an extremely fine matrix unless your scanner provides signal to burn (remember the drive to high field strength) or the indications warrant this added time.

One compromise commonly used is an asymmetric matrix such as 128 x 256. Increasing the matrix size in the frequency direction requires applying a stronger gradient that does not add time. In addition, using phase encoding for the short side of this rectangular matrix will take the same time as a scan with a128 x 128 matrix while still providing a finer detail.

In Figure A4.1, you probably noticed the artifacts of high signal intensity projected over the spinal canal. This is due to misregistration of the signal arising from flowing blood in the large pelvic blood vessels. Remember that motion on MR is always projected into the phase direction, which in this case runs craniocaudal. In Figure A4.2, look at the background noise behind the patient. See how it conforms to the contour of the anterior abdominal wall fat? Phase artifacts occur with any motion, not just vascular motion, and in this case we see the artifacts from the motion of the subcutaneous fat during respiration. The phase-encoding direction in Figure A4.2 is directed anterior to posterior, and therefore frequency encoding is craniocaudal. That explains why the inferior endplates are better seen (see Artifact 8).

While it is logical to choose the short side of a rectangular matrix for phase, it is helpful to match this matrix to the imaging problem based on logical guidelines. First, as is evident in Figure A4.1, the anticipated phase artifacts should not overlie the region of interest. It is also helpful to select the phase direction for the short side of the body part imaged. For example, for spine imaging, it makes sense to assign phase in the anterior-posterior direction since the human body is narrower in that dimension. With anterior-posterior phase encoding, slab saturation bands can be used effectively to suppress artifacts from the anterior abdominal wall.

Artifact 5

This 30-year-old postpartum woman presents with new headaches. Figure A5.1 is the maximum intensity projection (MIP) image from her coronal two-dimensional time-of-flight MR venogram (2D TOF MRV) using a saturation band in the neck that suppressed arterial flow. Your diagnosis is:

(1) superior sagittal sinus thrombosis.

(2) normal.

(3) superior sagittal sinus stenosis.

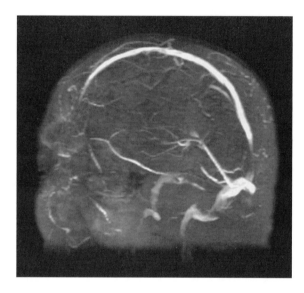

Figure A5.1

TIME-OF-FLIGHT MRA: IN-PLANE FLOW ARTIFACTS

Two-dimensional TOF imaging is an elegant and effective MRA technique that provides an accurate depiction of vascular structures without the need for any intravenous contrast. The contrast between the vascular lumen and the background is due entirely to entry slice enhancement of blood flow (see Artifact 1). Because the image is acquired as a stack of individual slices, every slice represents an entry slice for blood flow. A stack of thin images of the brain can then be transformed into MIP reconstructions that depict the intracranial venous system for example. While there are advantages to using a 2D TOF technique instead of 3D TOF , namely, sensitivity to relatively slow flow and almost unlimited coverage, there are some artifacts that have to be considered as a result of its single plane of acquisition.

Entry slice enhancement is most effective when the orientation of the acquisition slice is perpendicular to the direction of flow (Figures A5.2 and A5.3). For the cervical vasculature, this is ideal since flow in the vessels of interest is almost entirely directed toward the head. While this requirement limits its usefulness for intracranial arterial vessels that curve and loop, coronal 2D TOF is used for intracranial MRV because the venous flow in the brain is largely anterior to posterior and has relatively slow velocity compared with flow in cerebral arteries.

In Figure A5.1, you should have noticed that the superior sagittal sinus (SSS) is well demonstrated throughout with the exception of the posterior segment at its junction with the straight sinus at the torcula. While this appearance can be readily mistaken for intraluminal thrombus or stenosis, it is important to recognize that this is an artifact of *in- plane flow*. Since intravascular signal is highest when flow is perpendicular to the slice and lowest when flow is in the same plane as the slice, the signal in the SSS drops off in this vertical segment of the sinus that is in plane on a coronal acquisition. This effect is exaggerated in Figure A5.2, where the flow from the entire SSS drops off when the acquisition direction for the scan is turned to sagittal. It is important to know how the source data for the 2D TOF study were acquired in order to anticipate these artifacts (Figure A5.4 and A5.5). Acquiring two 2D TOF MRV scans in perpendicular directions or using contrast can help resolve some of the problems created by in-plane flow.

Correct answer: 2

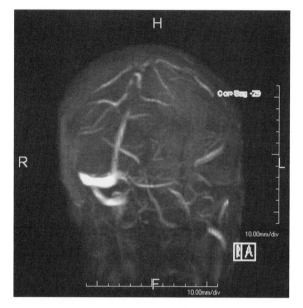

Figure A5.2

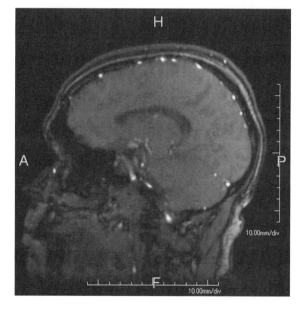

Figure A5.3

The acquisition plane for the 2D TOF scan used for the MIP image in Figure A5.2 was sagittal (Figure A5.3 is a source image from the scan), not coronal. That explains why this image appears so unusual. Where exactly are those cortical veins going? Nearly the entire superior sagittal sinus is absent because its flow is entirely in plane on this scan. The cortical veins are more apparent than on the usual coronal plane acquistion MRV because their flow is from lateral to medial and therefore perpendicular to this sagittal acquisition plane.

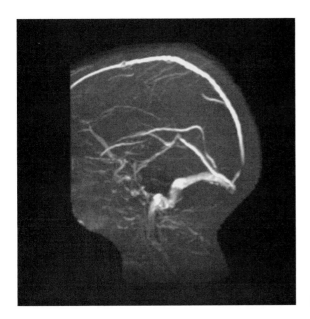

Figure A5.4

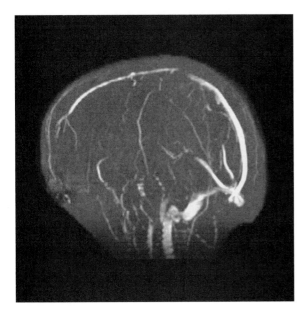

Figure A5.5

These two MRV scans were obtained one after the other. The 2D TOF MIP reconstruction from coronal scanning (Figure A5.4) demonstrates the expected signal dropout in the posterior SSS. The same 2D TOF sequence was repeated, but now with the acquisition slice orientation in the axial plane (Figure A5.5). Notice how the posterior sagittal sinus appears normal but there is now an apparent interruption in the middle of the SSS. This is due to another in-plane flow artifact but in a different location. You may also have noticed that the deep venous system is more apparent on the coronal acquisition (Figure A5.4). This is because the flow there is almost entirely from front to back, so coronal imaging is ideal to maximize that intravascular signal.

Artifact 6

This patient with colon cancer was called back after this MR scan (Figure A6.1) for a CT scan of the chest because of concern for pulmonary metastatic disease based on this MR scan. The CT scan will show:

(1) one lesion.

(2) two lesions.

(3) no lesions.

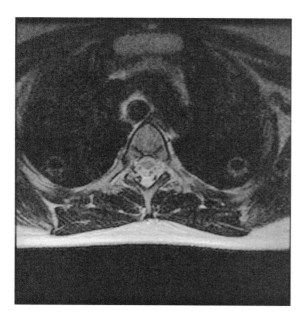

Figure A6.1

MOTION-RELATED GHOSTING ARTIFACTS

Blood vessels with high flow velocity, like the carotid artery, usually appear dark on MR images. This is due to signal losses caused by the turbulent flow leading to loss of phase coherence of the hydrogen spins. This effect is described as *intravoxel dephasing*. In many blood vessels we may be able to recover some signal, but this will have scrambled phase information due to movement between the applications of the gradients as well as turbulence, which also mixes the phases a bit. This leads to erroneous assignment of the location of their signal, much like a ventriloquist playing the game "Marco Polo." You may be familiar with this game, which is usually played in a swimming pool; one player closes his or her eyes and then must locate the other players using only the sound of their voices. When the seeker calls out "Marco," all the other players must respond "Polo."

The incorrect phase information, just as the ventriloquist misrepresents his or her location, then gets reconstructed at a distance from the source and can appear as a smear across the image or as discrete replicas of the structure called *ghosts*. These ghosts are particularly confusing when they vary in appearance, i.e., dark and bright (Figure A6.2). The bright ghosts are areas where the misplaced signal augments that of the tissue that should be there and the dark ghosts are the result of cancellation of this background tissue signal. It is important to be aware of this particular artifact so that this misplaced signal is not mistaken for a brain or liver lesion, for example (Figures A6.2 –A6.5).

Correct answer: 3

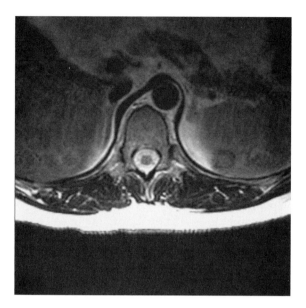

Figure A6.2 This T2WI demonstrates flow-related artifacts from the CSF flow displaced laterally, in the phase direction, from the spinal canal. Notice that the misplaced ghosts are both bright and dark.

In these enhanced MR scans, there is high-signal ghosting from venous flow that accounts for the apparently enhancing lesions in the brain. Do not mistake these ghosts for true parenchymal enhancement.

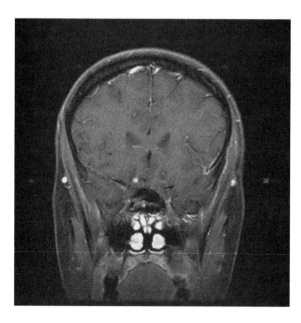

Figure A6.3

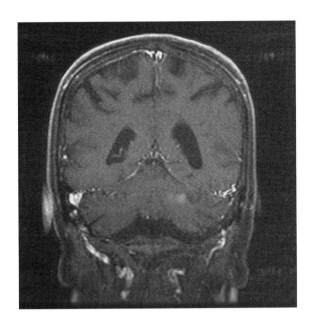

Figure A6.4

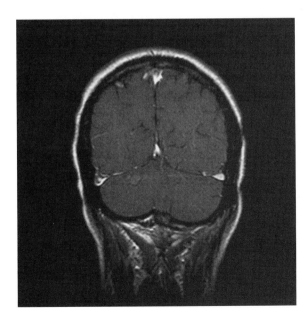

Figure A6.5

Artifact 7

This left-handed patient with a history of atherosclerotic disease presents with a history of dizziness when he plays tennis. His axial 2D TOF source image (Figure A7.1) along with the MIP reconstruction of the 2D TOF data (Figure A7.2) are provided, and you think they are consistent with the diagnosis of:

(1) subclavian steal.

(2) occlusion of the left vertebral artery.

(3) Either.

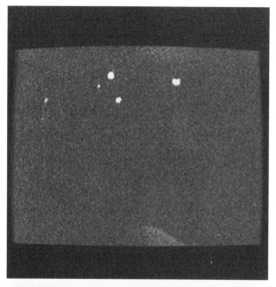

Figure A7.1

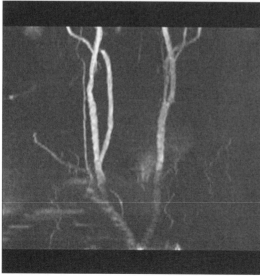

Figure A7.2

2D TOF DIRECTION OF FLOW ARTIFACTS

This case is a good example of how understanding the physics of MR imaging will allow you to better understand the limitations of MR techniques. While there appears to be flow in the common carotid arteries and a single vertebral artery, it would be more accurate to say that the Figure A7.1 demonstrates antegrade flow (caudal to cephalad) in both carotids and the right vertebral artery. That is because it would be incorrect to state that the left vertebral artery is occluded without more information.

The source images used for 2D TOF imaging are single slices acquired with the gradient echo technique. Since the image is a single slice, flow from either direction entering this slice will appear bright. You may wonder why we see only arteries, with no sign of the jugular veins on 2DTOF scans of the neck (Figures A7.3 and A7.4). The reason is that the individual slices are linked to a saturation band, called a *walking saturation band,* that moves together with the acquisition slice. This saturation band is designed to suppress signal from the hydrogen spins in that specific location. In order to see only arteries in the neck, that walking saturation band just needs to be positioned above the image acquisition slice. In that location, all signal from vessels flowing toward the feet, presumably veins, will be canceled, leaving just the bright entry slice enhancement from arterial flow that arrives from the opposite direction. If we reverse the position of the saturation band and put it above the image slice, the arteries will now be suppressed leaving only the signal arising from the veins (Figures A7.5 and A7.6).

As with many things in life, this elegant solution to the problem of selective arterial imaging can be both a blessing and a curse. The patient imaged in Figure A7.1 has what is called a *subclavian steal.* In this condition, the blood supply to the arm from the aorta is blocked by a proximal subclavian occlusion or stenosis, usually due to atherosclerotic disease (Figures A7.7 and A7.8). Because the vertebral arteries join together distally and connect with the subclavian arteries proximally, one can be recruited to supply blood flow to the involved arm by reversing its direction of flow. This is called a subclavian *steal* since the normal blood flow to the brain is diverted away from the brain. Since all flow in the cranial to caudal direction is suppressed on these 2D TOF images, this downward flow in the vertebral artery will be inapparent on standard 2D TOF imaging just as flowing blood the neck veins is suppressed.

To know definitely whether the vertebral artery is occluded, you would need to repeat the 2D TOF scan with the saturation band on the bottom of the acquisition slice, add a TOF exam in the neck without any saturation, or acquire a contrast-enhanced MRA scan. The last technique uses a rapid T1WI volume acquisition after injection of contrast. By injecting the contrast relatively rapidly and imaging when the contrast bolus arrives in the arteries, in the same fashion as for a computed tomographic angiography (CTA) scan, the enhanced blood will appear bright regardless of the direction of flow. In the contrast arch study of this patient (Figure A7.7), not only is there flow apparent in a good-sized left vertebral artery (arrow), but the subclavian artery that would ordinarily provide blood flow to the left arm is occluded just beyond its origin (arrowhead). From this image, we can conclude that the left vertebral artery is open but that flow in it has reversed in order to provide supply the left arm.

Correct answer: 3

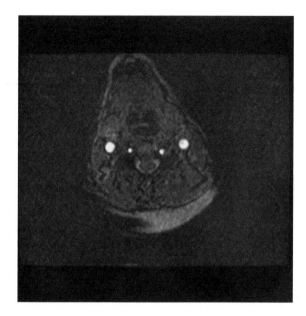

Figure A7.3

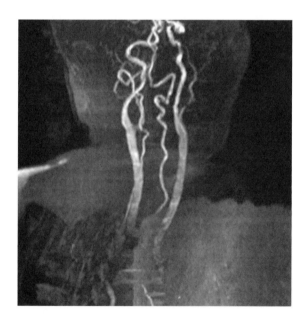

Figure A7.4

Figure A7.3 is a source image from the 2D TOF MRA of a different patient. On this exam a "walking" saturation band was placed on the cephalad side of the acquisition slice. This allows you to see the vertebral (arrow) and carotid arteries (arrowhead) without veins, since their signal is suppressed, on the source image and then, of course, on the reconstructed MIP (Figure A7.4).

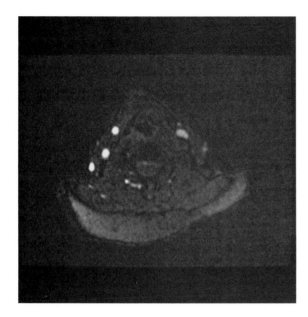

Figure A7.5

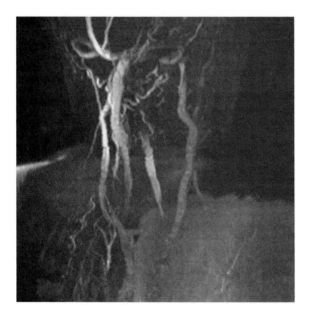

Figure A7.6

If we do exactly the same 2D TOF acquisition as seen in Figure A7.3 but place the saturation band on the caudal (i.e. opposite) side of the acquisition slice, we now see only blood flow directed towards the feet. Now there will be no signal from the usual arterial flow, that is nearly all directed towards the head. Based on their location in the neck on the acquisition slice (Figure A7.5) these bright vessels are the neck veins, not arteries. By changing the position of the saturation band an image of the neck veins, can be created (Figure A7.6) using the 2DTOF technique.

This reliance on direction of flow with 2D TOF imaging can be problematic whenever imaging the carotid artery since this artery may have large vascular loops. While a flow gap in the carotid usually indicates a hemodynamically significant stenosis, you may also see a gap whenever the direction of flow in the carotid reverses in a loop (Figures A7.9 and A7.10).

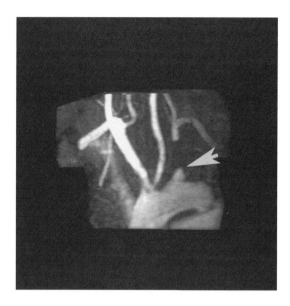

Figure A7.7

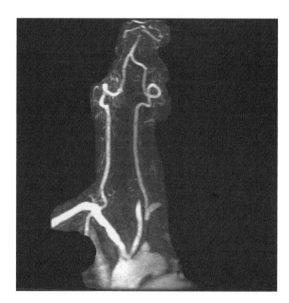

Figure A7.8

Figure A7.7 from a contrast enhanced volume acquisition shows the expected vascular anatomy at the aortic arch associated with subclavian steal. This patient most likely had a long-standing left subclavian occlusion from atherosclerotic disease. The flow in the left vertebral artery has reversed in order to provide blood flow to the left arm, which is well depicted in the segmented image of Figure A7.8, where you can see the connection between the right vertebral artery and left subclavian artery via the vertebrobasilar junction.

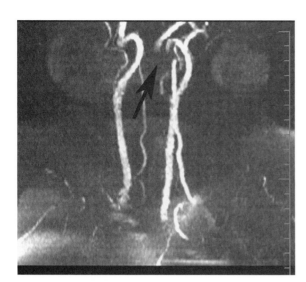

Figure A7.9

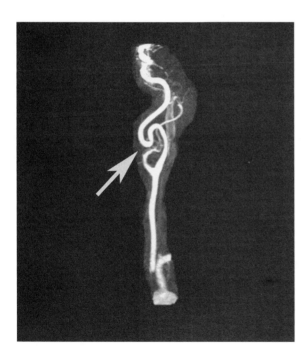

Figure A7.10

The walking saturation band is designed to suppress venous flow but it is not selective for veins, only for direction of flow. If the carotid has a large downward loop (arrow in Figure A7.9), this downward arterial flow will also be suppressed resulting in a gap in the vessel. The advantage of using a contrast enhanced MRA technique (Figure A7.10) is that it will show a complete loop (arrow); since it does not rely on flow related enhancement, it is insensitive to the direction of blood flow.

Artifact 8

This 25-year-old female was in a terrible rollover motor vehicle accident late one snowy night. She has an obvious spine fracture on CT (Figure A8.1), but you are called in at 2 a.m. because the surgeons want to operate immediately based on the MR finding of what is believed to be an acute intraspinal hemorrhage on T1WI (Figure A8.2) and T2WI (Figure A8.3). After a careful review of the images you decide that:

(1) this must be an old hemorrhage.

(2) she has an acute hemorrhage.

(3) this is not blood at all.

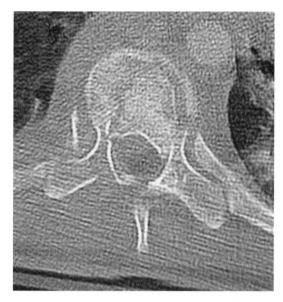

Figure A8.1

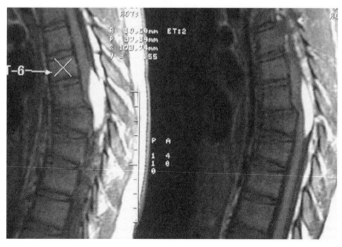

Figure A8.2

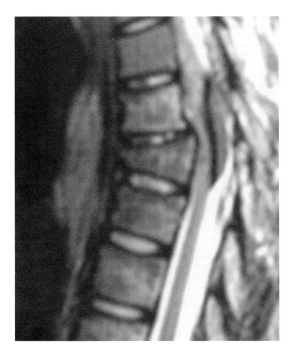

Figure A8.3

CHEMICAL SHIFT ARTIFACTS

The chemical shift artifact on the MR images in this case was an important clue to the correct diagnosis (Figure A8.3). Chemical shift artifacts can occur whenever there is an interface between fat and watery tissues. It always is visible in the frequency direction and never in the phase direction, which should be kept in mind whenever you consider this diagnosis. It is due to the slight difference between the Larmor frequency of hydrogen spins bound in fat and those bound in water. This difference is about 220 Hz on a 1.5 T scanner, a fairly small change considering that the Larmor frequency of water is 64 MHz at that field strength, but it is still enough to provide a visible displacement on MR images.

Remember that one axis of spatial location is based on frequency, so the position in that direction is determined by whether the returning signal has a low or high frequency. Because the hydrogen spins in fat are assigned the "wrong" location based on this frequency shift, a dark edge will appear on one side and a bright line will be evident on the other at a location where the water and fat signals overlap. Both the dark and bright borders may not necessarily be evident on the left side of the lipoma, however, since their conspicuity depends on the background signal. For example, only the dark border is evident in Figure A8.3.

Correct answer: 3. Chemical shift artifact from an incidental intraspinal lipoma.

There was very little question of the correct diagnosis when the CT scan was carefully reconsidered in light of the MR findings (Figure A8.4).

On many scans the chemical shift effects may be very evident or quite subtle, and a trained eye may be required to pick them out (Figures A8.5–A8.7). For example, notice on the sagittal gradient echo scan (Figure A8.8) that the lower vertebral end plates are quite distinct, while the upper end plates are not. This is another chemical shift effect that is the result of the cranial-caudal shift in frequency from fat within the bone marrow.

There are several approaches to minimizing chemical shift artifacts. One effective method is to do away with the fat signal altogether using a chemical fat suppression technique (Figures A8.9–A8.11).

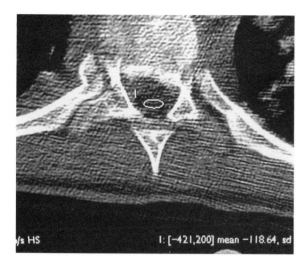

Figure A8.4 A cursor placed over the posterior spinal canal was characteristic for fat with an attenuation of HU-118.

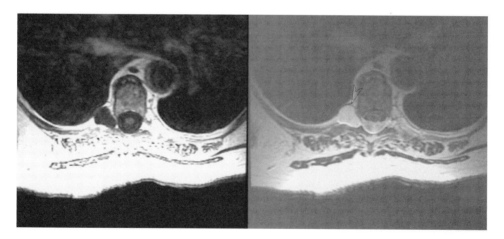

Figure A8.5 These axial images also demonstrate the characteristic appearance of chemical shift artifacts with a bright line at the posterior margin and a dark line at the anterior edge of this root sleeve cyst due to the displacement of signal at the fat-water interface (arrowhead in the right image of Figure A8.5).

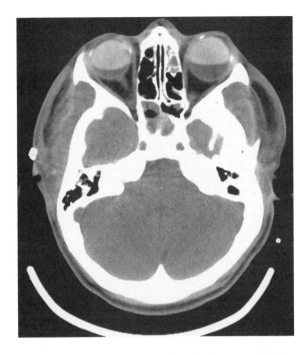

Figure A8.6

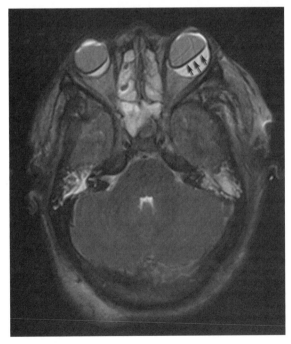

Figure A8.7

This patient had an intraocular silicone injection for retinal detachment, seen here on CT (Figure A8.6). Note the striking chemical shift artifacts (arrows) on the T2WI (Figure A8.7). Silicone provides an even larger chemical shift with water than fat, which explains the conspicuity of the artifact in this case.

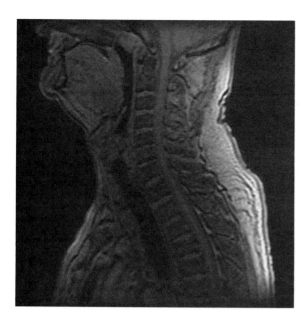

Figure A8.8 If you look carefully, you can see that the inferior end plates of these vertebral bodies are much better defined than the superior end plates. This is the result of chemical shift artifact in the frequency direction between the water and fat components in the bone marrow. Since the phase direction is usually anterior to posterior to minimize flow as well as wraparound artifacts, frequency encoding (and therefore chemical shift) is in the cranial-caudal direction on most spine images.

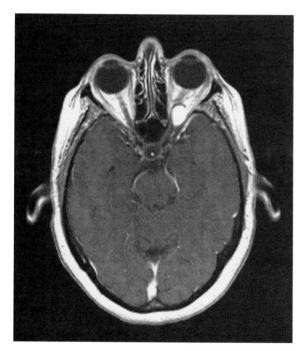

Figure A8.9

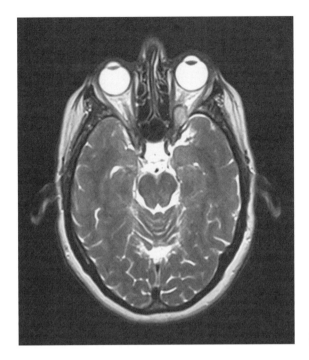

Figure A8.10

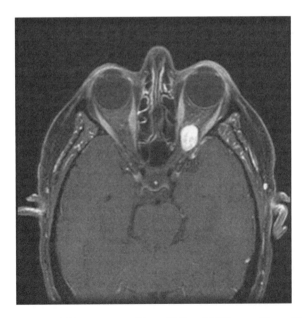

Figure A8.11

The axial T1WI postcontrast (Figure A8.9) and T2WI scans (Figure A8.10) both demonstrate a dark line at the anterior border of this intraorbital mass. On the other postcontrast T1WI scan (Figure A8.11), there is no chemical shift artifact because the fat signal has been suppressed using a chemical fat suppression technique.

Artifact 9

This 35-year-old woman presented with left-sided facial pain. Her physician ordered an MR scan with contrast to determine the source of the pain, and she was scheduled in the first outpatient slot one week later. Your partner is reading the MR scan that day, notes abnormal signal in the left orbit on both the enhanced coronal and axial T1WI scans (Figures A9.1 and A9.2), and calls the patient's physician. They are both puzzled, however, because the patient's pain had resolved during the interval between her presentation and her MR scan.

As they are talking about the case, you comment on this nice example of:

(1) chemical shift artifact.

(2) lymphoma.

(3) incomplete fat saturation.

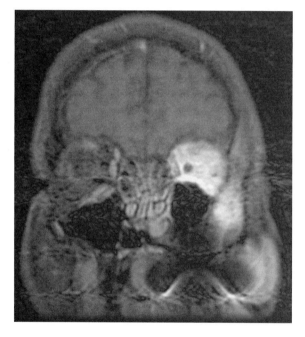

Figure A9.1

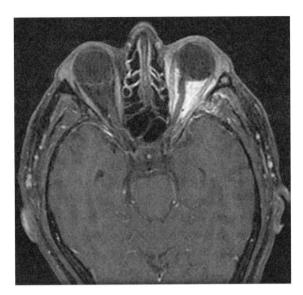

Figure A9.2

CHEMICAL FAT SUPPRESSION AND STIR ARTIFACTS

There are several ways to suppress the signal from fat on MR. STIR is a very useful technique that suppresses fat signal by using an inversion pulse followed by a 90 degree pulse at the precise time that the net magnetization of short T1 tissue like fat crosses the zero axis. While STIR is frequently used for spine and extremity imaging, it is not well suited to imaging with contrast because it suppresses fat and enhancing tissues equally well. This is because STIR suppresses any tissue with short T1 relaxation time.

Chemical fat suppression is a technique designed to suppress only fat signal. While it is ideal for imaging enhancement within the fat in cases of orbital masses or soft tissue tumors, reliable chemical fat suppression puts a premium on the homogeneity of the magnetic field. This often proves to be a limiting factor since the magnetic field is frequently inhomogeneous, particularly at the periphery of the bore or edge of a surface coil.

The chemical fat suppression sequence uses a precise presaturation pulse tuned to the frequency of fat, a technique based on the principle that hydrogen spins bound in fat precess at a slightly different frequency than hydrogen spins bound in water (see Artifact 8). By applying this prepulse at the precise Larmor frequency of fat and then scrambling the phase of the resulting signal, fat becomes invisible on the image. If everything goes as planned, nearly all of the signal recovered on the scan, regardless of whether that scan is T1 or T2 weighted, will come from nonfat hydrogen spins.

This is ideal for contrast-enhanced T1 imaging because enhancing tissue will appear more conspicuous against a dark background. In practice, however, it is possible to mistake poor suppression for enhancement if anything distorts the homogeneity of the magnetic field and interferes with optimal suppression (Figures A9.3–A9.6).

Correct answer: 3

You may wonder, why bother? The reason is that without chemical fat suppression, it is possible for abnormal enhancing tissue in the eye or spine to be overlooked on postcontrast T1WI. This is because the high signal from contrast enhancement may allow the tumor to match that of the background fat. In this way it is possible to make a tumor, otherwise easily visible on the noncontrast scan, disappear on the postcontrast scan. This is why you should avoid reading enhanced-only T1 images of the spine (Figures A9.7 and A9.8).

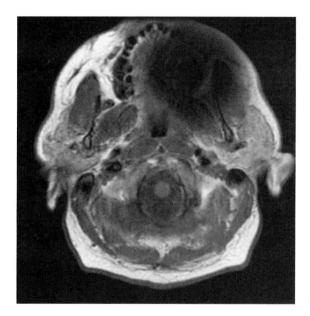

Figure A9.3 The T1WI axial scan at a lower level (Figure A9.3) demonstrates the large artifact arising from dental metal that distorts the magnetic field in the orbit sufficiently to degrade the quality of fat suppression in the left orbit that was evident in Figures A9.1 and A9.2.

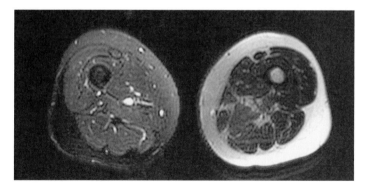

Figure A9.4 This T1WI that includes the left and right thighs was obtained with chemical fat suppression. The two legs look completely different because the patient's left leg was off center in the scanner. This degraded the quality of fat suppression due to magnetic field inhomogeneities in the peripheral magnetic field. (Image provided by Douglas Goodwin, MD, Dartmouth-Hitchcock Medical Center, Lebanon, NH.)

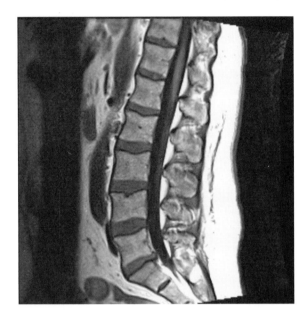

Figure A9.5

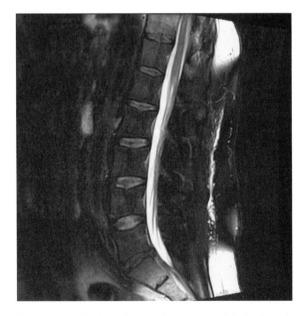

Figure A9.6

This sagittal T1WI shows the normal appearance of the lumbar spine and soft tissues (Figure A9.5). The T2WI with fat suppression (Figure A9.6) shows what appears to be increased marrow signal in the sacrum and lower thoracic spine because there is good fat suppression in the midlumbar region but no fat suppression in the subcutaneous fat in the upper and lower back. This is because the fat suppression is incomplete at the ends of this surface coil which is positioned directly over the patient's midlumbar spine. This effect may also be evident on sagittal, large field of view images in short bore magnets because of the inhomogeneity of the magnetic field at the ends of the bore.

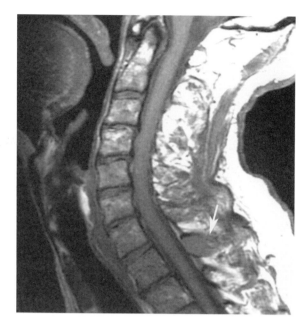

Figure A9.7

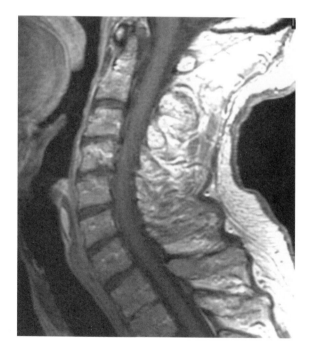

Figure A9.8

The sagittal T1WI (Figure A9.7) demonstrates a low-signal metastatic lesion involving the body and spinous process of T1 (arrow). On the postcontrast T1WI scan (Figure A9.8), it is much less conspicuous because the contrast shortens T1 to the point where the diseased marrow space appears similar in signal to the normal fatty marrow at other levels.

Artifact 10

This patient had a postoperative scan immediately after posterior fossa surgery because of mental status changes. While the brain appeared normal, there were two signal voids in the Sylvian fissures suggesting middle cerebral artery (MCA) aneurysms on the T2WI (Figure A10.1, arrows). The signal voids were also evident on the T1WI (Figure A10.2) and diffusion scans (Figure A10.3). Based on these findings you think this patient has:

(1) bilateral subarachnoid hemorrhages.

(2) bilateral MCA aneurysms.

(3) neither.

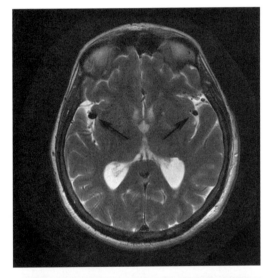

Figure A10.1

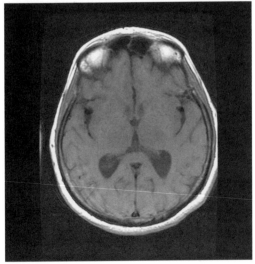

Figure A10.2

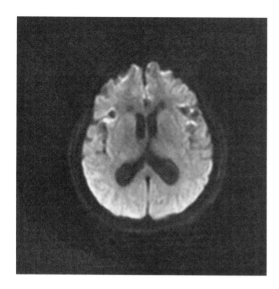

Figure A10.3

FLOW AND SUSCEPTIBILITY

This case illustrates in a nutshell the difference between reading a CT scan, where there is a linear relationship between pixel intensity and its attenuation of X-rays, and an MR scan, where there is usually more than one reason that a pixel is dark or bright (Figure A10.4). A signal void, like those on T2WI (Figure A10.1), could be due to low proton density, short T2 relaxation time, susceptibility, or flow. In this particular location, it is hard to get past the notion that the patient has two aneurysms. However, the bright rim evident on the diffusion scan (Figure A10.3) indicates susceptibility effects that would not be expected in association with an aneurysm (Figures A10.5 and A10.6).

This is a good time to introduce the terms *permeability* and *susceptibility*. Some materials, like iron, are described as having a very high magnetic *permeability* because magnetic flux lines will go out of their way to go through iron . As a result these ordinarily evenly distributed flux lines are displaced and become more compact within ferromagnetic metals. This propensity to have a very high *flux density* is the reason it is advantageous to make an electromagnet with an iron core. This concept is also relevant to any discussion of how the fringe field from a large scanner magnet is modified, or shielded, by large plates of iron. In that situation the magnetic flux lines that otherwise would extend far beyond the magnet are constrained by surrounding the magnet with iron plates. This is because these field lines will compact within the iron because of its high magnetic permeability, leading to lower flux density beyond the confines of the metal shielding. This property of ferromagnetic materials can also be described in a relative way using the term magnetic *susceptibility*, using air as a reference with a value of 1. While ferromagnetic metals have susceptibility values greater than 1, most tissues in the body are *diamagnetic* and have values less than 1. These diamagnetic materials have just the opposite interaction with magnetism and so the flux lines behave as though they would prefer to be elsewhere.

Correct answer: 3. This represents post-operative intracranial air.

These differences in susceptibility, while still quite small for air and brain, are sufficient to distort the homogeneity of the scanner's magnetic field and in that way become evident on some pulse sequences. While not visible on FSE-T2WI, there is usually enough distortion to be visible on echoplanar diffusion, T2* gradient sequences, and certainly on susceptibility weighted imaging (SWI). Because of the considerable difference in susceptibility between brain and even paramagnetic metals such as those used in aneurysm clips, some artifacts will be evident on all MR pulse sequences.

It is important to keep in mind the relative sensitivities of the different pulse sequences when looking for and identifying susceptibility artifacts. If there is a question of intracranial cavernomas, for example, a scan sensitive to susceptibility effects might be added for that patient exam (Figures A10.7–A10.10). A relatively new pulse sequence called *susceptibility-weighted imaging* (SWI) is so sensitive that it can even demonstrate differences in blood vessels due to their levels of oxygenation of hemoglobin.

Figure A10.11 demonstrates another very common susceptibility artifact, this time due to eye makeup. The pigments in eye shadow and eye liner may include iron that distorts the magnetic field sufficiently to alter the anterior contour of the eyes. This is ordinarily just a nuisance, but it can degrade the quality of orbit images, so patients should be advised to arrive for their orbit MR scan without eye makeup. In patients with permanent eye liner tattoos, this may cause heating during the MR scan sufficient to be a source of discomfort, but it is not a contraindication for an MR scan since reactions are rare and minor. You should be aware that skin tattoos anywhere on the body have the potential to heat up, depending on the pigments, the location of the tattoo, and the type of imaging coil. Keep this in mind if patients complain of symptoms in the region of tattoos during or after their scan.

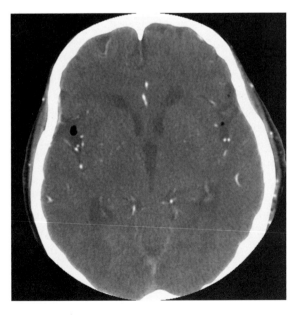

Figure A10.4 This axial CT scan with contrast nicely demonstrates that the signal voids on MR were due to intracranial air and not flow.

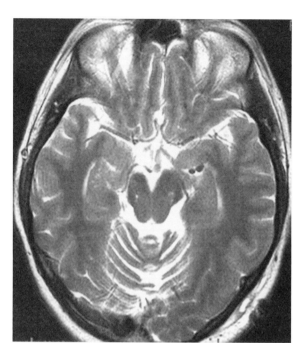

Figure A10.5

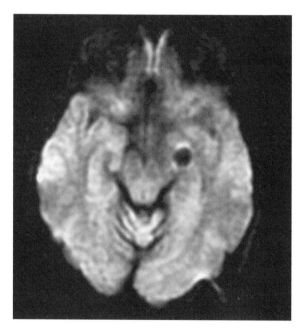

Figure A10.6

The T2WI (Figure A10.5) is another example of a signal void from intracranial air, this time intraventricular. The diffusion scan (Figure A10.6) also demonstrates central low signal but with peripheral high signal typical of susceptibility artifacts.

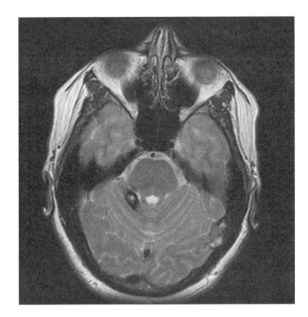

Figure A10.7

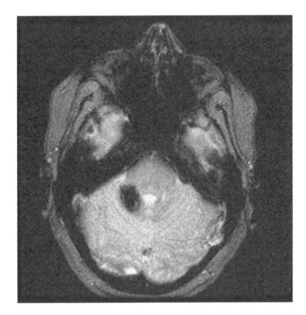

Figure A10.8

In this example, the susceptibility artifact around the cerebellar cavernoma is smaller on the T2 FSE image (Figure A10.7) than on the gradient echo scan (Figure A10.8).This enlargement, called *blooming*, helps to differentiate flow from susceptibility artifact since the size of the signal void from flow should remain the same on all sequences.

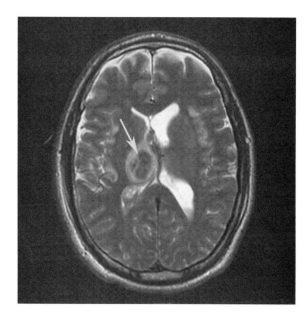

Figure A10.9

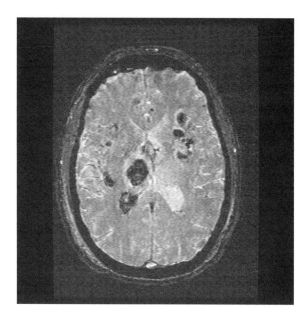

Figure A10.10

The T2 FSE image (Figure A10.9) shows abnormal signal from a traumatic hemorrhage in the right thalamus (arrow). On a more susceptibility-weighted scan (Figure A10.10), you can characterize this as blood based on the signal dropout from susceptibility effects in the thalamus as well as the left and right sylvian fissures and ventricle.

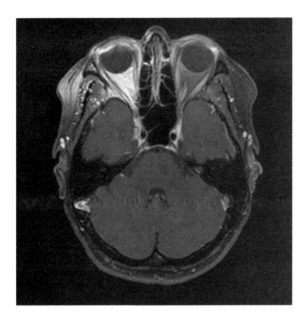

Figure A10.11 On this axial T1WI fat-suppressed scan, note the flattened anterior contour of the globes, which is due entirely to distortion of the magnetic field from eye makeup.

Artifact 11

These T1 axial postcontrast MR images of the pelvis were obtained in two different patients. While there is the expected high signal visible within the bladder on both scans as a result of the T1 effects of IV contrast excretion in urine, how would you account for the unusual distribution of contrast in Figure A11.1?

(1) There is a mass in the bladder.

(2) There is blood layering in the dependent part of the bladder.

(3) T2 effects of contrast.

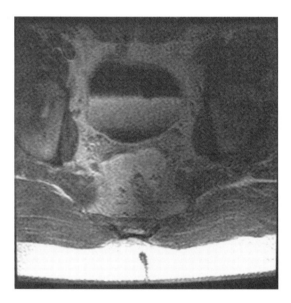

Figure A11.1

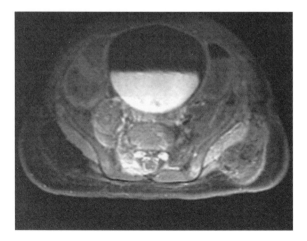

Figure A11.2

T2 EFFECTS OF CONTRAST AND THE PARFAIT SIGN

This finding I like to call the *parfait sign* since it reminds me of those desserts that consist of layers of ice cream and syrup served in a tall glass. In this instance, the layers we see in the bladder (Figure A11.1) provide an important illustration of the differences between iodinated and gadolinium contrast agents. Let's consider the top layer in the bladders first. Magnetic resonance contrast, like iodinated contrast used for CT, is denser than urine. Therefore, we should expect clear urine at the top layer, so the low signal there is due to the expected long T1 of water. The high signal within both bladders indicates where the contrast and urine have mixed to the degree that we see the T1 effects that make urine appear bright on a T1WI. The bladder in Figure A11.2 looks about the same way a contrast-enhanced bladder appears on CT. This is because MR and CT intravenous contrast agents have much in common. For example, both iodine and gadolinium are bound to large molecules, both accumulate wherever there is an interruption in the blood-brain barrier in the brain, and both are largely cleared by the kidneys and excreted in urine.

There is, however, one very important difference between the two. Iodine provides contrast on CT simply by providing increased attenuation of X-rays compared with the soft tissues of the body like brain or liver. The nature of this effect is linear and quite predictable. That is, the higher the concentration of iodine, the higher the attenuation of the X-ray beam to the point that at a very high concentration, streak artifacts become evident due to photon starvation, much like the artifacts from metal on CT. As a result, contrast on CT appears white, while low-attenuation tissue like fat or urine appears black.

The effect of gadolinium, on the other hand, is visible only indirectly as a result of the way it speeds up the relaxation of nearby hydrogen protons, which shortens their T1 relaxation times. We are very familiar with this T1 shortening effect since, at the concentrations seen in soft tissue tumors, this is the only visible effect. It is not as widely appreciated that gadolinium contrast also shortens T2 relaxation times, however, because this effect is evident only when its concentration is quite high. Because of the renal excretion of contrast these high concentrations of gadolinium are commonly encountered in the renal collecting system and bladder.

Correct answer: 3

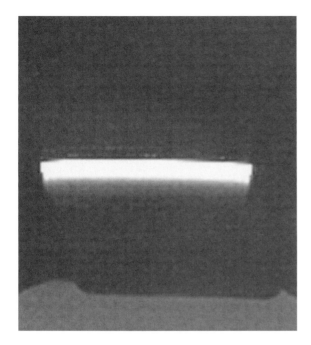

Figure A11.3

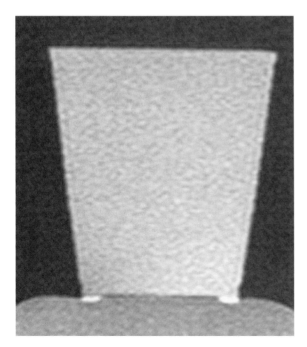

Figure A11.4

The T1WI (Figure A11.3) shows the bright interface between the layers of high-concentration gadolinium below and enhanced water above. The T1WI image (Figure A11.4) shows the cup after mixing in more water, with the contrast lowering the concentration of gadolinium to the point where T1 effects of the contrast predominate.

Since the highest concentrations of contrast might be expected in the most dependent portion of the bladder, T2 shortening alone readily explains why the lower layer of the bladder in Figure A11.1 is dark. While it does appear similar to the top layer in the bladder, remember that there is always more than one source of contrast on MR images. We can also think of this relationship between contrast and water like the porridge in the story "Goldilocks and the Three Bears." The different layers in the bladder reflect too little contrast at the top, too much at the bottom, and "just right" in the middle.

If you are still skeptical, look at these images of a Styrofoam cup filled with water (Figure A11.3). On this image, taken after gadolinium contrast was slowly added to water in the cup, you can see a bright band where the concentration is "just right" for T1 relaxation enhancement and low signal is apparent at the bottom, where the T2 effects of the contrast predominate. After adding some more water and mixing it up, the dilute contrast is now distributed evenly throughout the cup and the water becomes uniformly bright due to the expected gadolinium T1 effects (Figure A11.4). This effect is again evident in the extrarenal pelvis of the left kidney in this patient where you can see two parallel fluid levels (Figure A11.5).

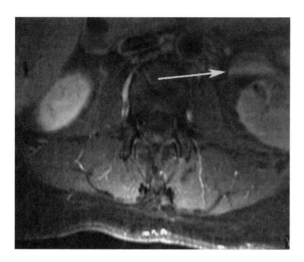

Figure A11.5 This is an example of the parfait effect in the left renal collecting system (arrow), where the high concentration of contrast in the dependent portion of this extrarenal pelvis makes it appear dark on the fat-suppressed T1WI.

Artifact 12

This 73-year-old patient presents with new dizziness. The MR FLAIR scan (Figure A12.1) shows high signal in the asymmetric, widened left cerebellopontine angle (CPA) cistern. After reviewing the postcontrast T1 (Figure A12.2), diffusion (Figure A12.3), and T2-weighted images (Figure A12.4), you decide that the patient has:

(1) an epidermoid tumor.

(2) an arachnoid cyst.

(3) a cystic schwannoma.

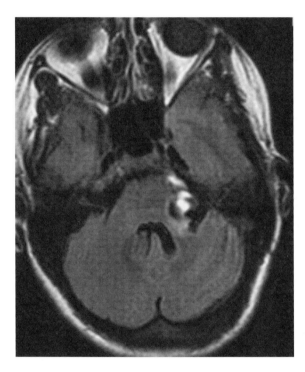

Figure A12.1

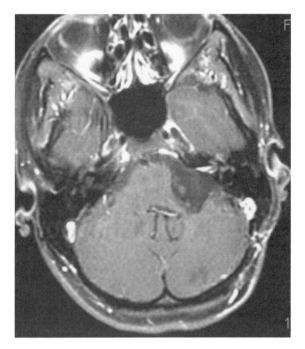

Figure A12.2

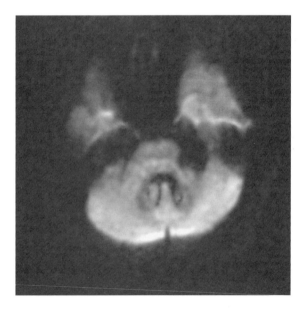

Figure A12.3

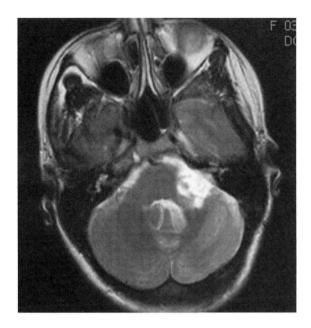

Figure A12.4

FLAIR FLOW ARTIFACTS

No tumor is evident on these scans. The findings are due to a CPA arachnoid cyst with flow from pulsations apparent on the FLAIR scan. Even though FLAIR images are inherently T2 weighted images, CSF should appear dark on FLAIR because the timing of the RF pulses used for this MR technique results in suppression of CSF. Because this is an IR sequence, by waiting several seconds to apply the 90 degree pulse (TI = 2200 msec), it occurs at the precise point in time when CSF net magnetization is passing the zero axis in its recovery path. Since there are no available spins to provide signal, normal CSF effectively disappears on FLAIR. The nearby brain or spinal cord will, of course, recover more quickly than CSF, so at the moment of the 90 degree pulse at 2200 msec, they would have many available hydrogen spins to provide signal.

When anything is added to the CSF, such as blood or protein, the hydrogen spins in CSF will recover more quickly than normal CSF. In that circumstance, the hydrogen spins in the abnormal CSF will recover beyond the zero point and therefore will be available to provide signal that appears brighter than the normal CSF. This exquisite sensitivity to factors that alter the character of CSF makes FLAIR a very powerful imaging sequence for the subarachnoid space (Figure A12.5).

Returning to Figure A12.1, why would flow alone result in increased signal from the otherwise normal CSF in the left CPA cistern? In order to suppress the signal from CSF, the hydrogen spins must experience the 180 and 90 degree pulses at a precise times. As a result of CSF flow, however, there may be sufficient movement of CSF to throw this timing off. Another potential cause for these FLAIR artifacts, which are particularly evident in the posterior fossa in general, is inhomogeneity of

Correct answer: 2

the magnetic field, either intrinsic or due to metal nearby. In any event, these artifacts limit the use of FLAIR for evaluation of the subarachnoid space below the tentorium for subarachnoid hemorrhage and create a variety of artifactual intraventricular lesions as well (Figures A12.6 and A12.7). While it was reasonable to consider an epidermoid or cystic tumor in this case based on the FLAIR findings, the normal diffusion scan and lack of enhancement on the other sequences make them unlikely.

How can you know when a wide CP angle cistern is due to an epidermoid and not a FLAIR flow artifact? Look at the diffusion scan (Figures A12.8–A12.10). Contrast images are helpful whenever there is increased signal on the FLAIR scan in a CSF space and tumor is a consideration (Figures A12.11 and A12.12).

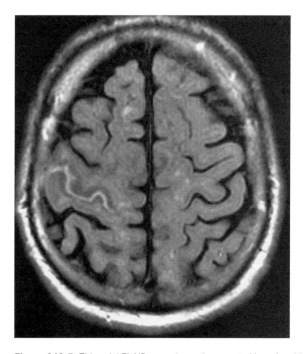

Figure A12.5 This axial FLAIR scan shows the expected low signal in all the cortical sulci except the right precentral sulcus, which is filled with blood in this patient with a small sudbarachnoid hemorrhage. Since hydrogen spins in the blood-CSF mix recover faster than protons in normal CSF elsewhere (shorter T1 relaxation time), they will provide relatively high signal when the 90 degree pulse is applied at a TI of 2200 msec.

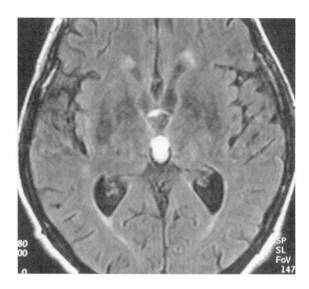

Figure A12.6

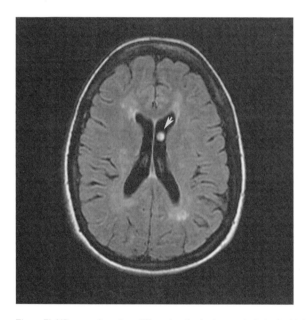

Figure A12.7

These FLAIR scans from two different patients demonstrate typical intraventricular FLAIR flow artifacts. What appears to be a rounded mass in the third ventricle (Figure A12.6) and the left lateral ventricle (arrow, Figure A12.7) is due pulsations of CSF.

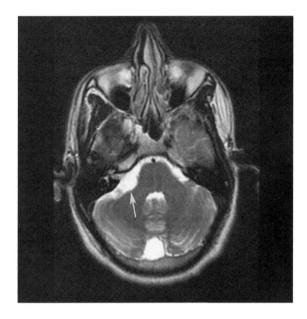

Figure A12.8

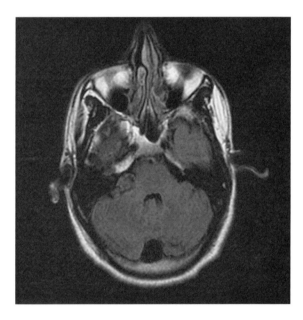

Figure A12.9

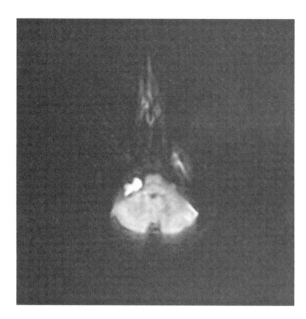

Figure A12.10

This patient also had a wide CPA cistern, well seen on the T2 scan (arrow, Figure A12.8). The FLAIR scan (Figure A12.9) also shows unsuppressed CSF in the CPA cistern compared with the fourth ventricle and cisterna magna. While this can also be due to flow, the hyperintensity on DWI in the same location (Figure A12.10) establishes the diagnosis of an epidermoid tumor instead of an arachnoid cyst or wide subarachnoid space.

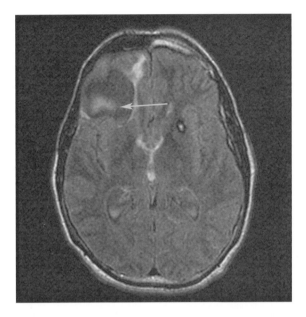

Figure A12.11

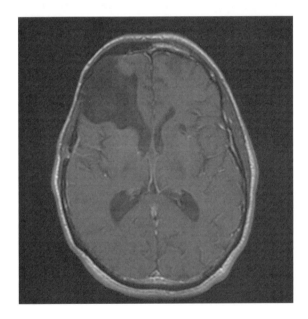

Figure A12.12

The axial FLAIR scan (Figure A12.11) in this patient who had a right frontal resection of a brain tumor demonstrates high signal in the posterior aspect of the cavity (arrow). This is due entirely to CSF flow within the large CSF space and not recurrent tumor, which is confirmed by the contrast-enhanced T1WI (Figure A12.12).

Artifact 13

This patient has a history of multiple sclerosis (MS), and you have an MR scan report from another hospital of a lesion in the middle cerebellar peduncle. A more recent FLAIR scan (Figure A13.1) at the appropriate level shows no abnormality. Is this most likely due to:

(1) treatment effects?

(2) insensitivity of FLAIR?

(3) the wrong diagnosis?

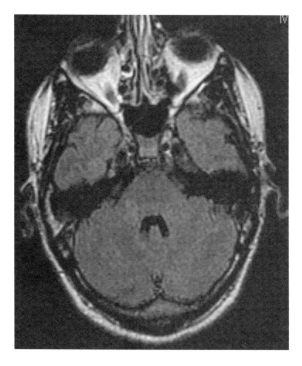

Figure A13.1

INFRATENTORIAL INSENSITIVITY OF FLAIR AND RELATIVE VALUE OF PULSE SEQUENCES

You may have noted some inhomgeneous signal in the right brachium pontis on Figure A13.1, but consider how much more confident you would have felt about your diagnosis had you seen the proton density sequence from the same MR examination (Figure A13.2, arrow).

It is not entirely clear why MS lesions below the tentorium are not well visualized on FLAIR, but this may be part of the same difficulties reported in finding MS lesions in the spinal cord using FLAIR. This case illustrates the value of knowing how to assign relative value to information from different MR scans. This becomes important when you have to reconcile conflicting evidence from two different sequences. In this instance, a lesion is visible on the proton density scan but not on the FLAIR scan, so you might argue that it a 50–50 decision. In practice, you should put a much higher value on the proton density scan in the posterior fossa once you recognize this limitation of FLAIR (Figures A13.3–A13.5). You probably use differential weighting of information in other aspects of your life. For example, you might undervalue a favorable review of a new movie provided by a friend who always enjoys movies that you hate. You have to consider the quality of the information when making decisions.

Another common example of this relative weighting of information is provided by postcontrast scans. It is not unusual to find that a lesion is faintly visible on a coronal scan but not at all visible on an axial scan. If you are not certain which scan to believe when confronted by this conflicting information, check the order of scanning. If the coronal scan was obtained after the axial scan, as is common, the additional time that elapsed after contrast injection usually makes the coronal scan more sensitive. This happens because, during that additional time, more contrast would have accumulated in the lesion through the interrupted blood-brain barrier.

You also need to know which pulse sequences are more sensitive to contrast enhancement itself. For detection of contrast enhancement, T1WI using spin echo is more sensitive than a gradient echo technique like spoiled gradient recalled (SPGR) and fat-suppressed T1WI is more sensitive than both (Figures A13.6 and A13.7). This is because the fat suppression pulse provides some magnetization transfer contrast effects to the image, which makes the contrast more conspicuous.

Correct answer: 2

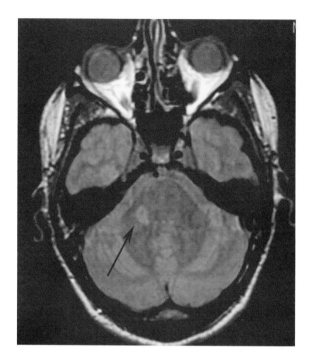

Figure A13.2 The proton density scan (Figure A13.2) clearly shows a lesion in the right brachium pontis (arrow) that was inapparent on the FLAIR scan (Figure A13.1).

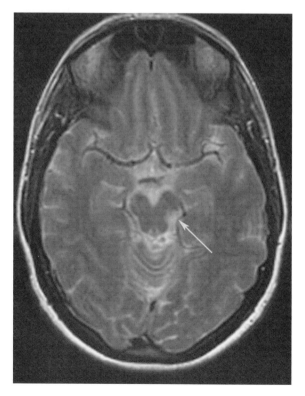

Figure A13.3

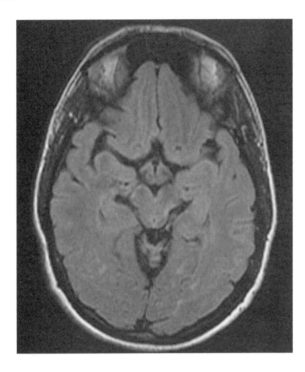

Figure A13.4

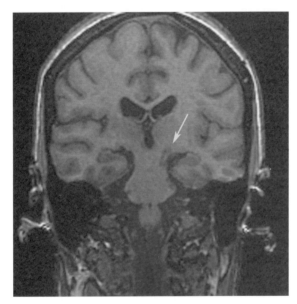

Figure A13.5

The axial T2WI (Figure A13.3) better demonstrates the lesion in the left midbrain (arrow) than the FLAIR scan (Figure A13.4) at the same level. If you need a tie breaker, this MS lesion was also evident on the coronal T1WI (Figure A13.5, arrow).

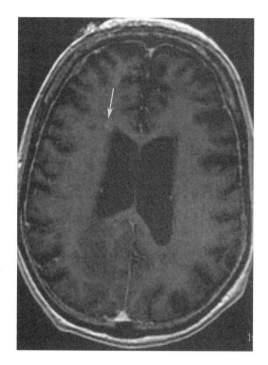

Figure A13.6

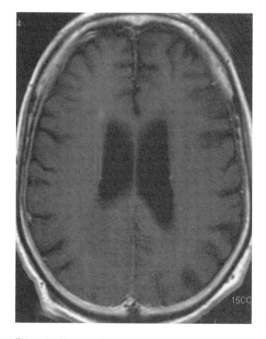

Figure A13.7

This pair of images illustrates one general principle of pulse sequence sensitivity to contrast. Compare the conspicuity of this metastatic lesion in the right frontal lobe on the gradient echo scan (arrow, Figure A13.6) to the conspicuity on the conventional spin echo T1WI scan (Figure A13.7), where the lesion is more apparent.

Artifact 14

This axial FLAIR scan (Figure A14.1) shows a large hemorrhage, but where is it located?

   (1) prepontine cistern.

   (2) fourth ventricle.

   (3) middle cerebellar peduncle.

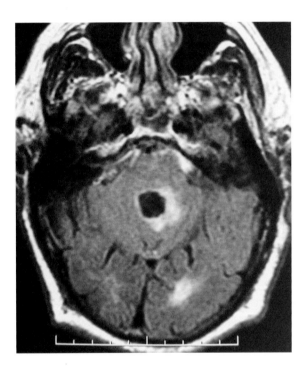

Figure A14.1

FLAIR AND ACUTE HEMORRHAGE

In this particular situation, a FLAIR scan can be difficult to interpret without using information from other sequences, and it illustrates the danger of forming opinions based on the findings from only one MR pulse sequence. In this example there is acute intraventricular hemorrhage inside the fourth ventricle, but because of the T2 effects of acute blood it appears dark––precisely how the suppressed CSF is expected to appear on FLAIR. The corresponding T2-weighted image (Figure A14.2) provides contrast between the blood and CSF because on that scan the normal CSF appears bright, while the blood remains dark. If you wondered about the signal in the prepontine cistern in Figure A14.1, that is due to unsuppressed CSF signal from flow (See Artifact 12). It is important to recognize that there is more than one source of contrast on FLAIR images, as on all MR imaging, so low signal is not necessarily due to CSF suppression alone. This is an important reason why you must consider the appearance of any focal finding across all the available pulse sequences (Figures A14.3–A14.6).

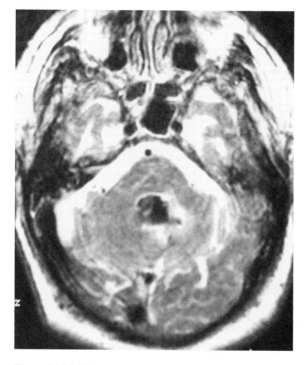

Figure A14.2 This axial T2WI at the same level as Figure A14.1, demonstrates abnormal low signal in the fourth ventricle due to the T2 effects of acute hemorrhage. This blood is inapparent on the FLAIR scan (Figure A14.1) because the low signal from T2 effects of the blood closely matches the expected low signal of normal CSF due to the suppression of CSF signal on FLAIR.

Correct answer: 2

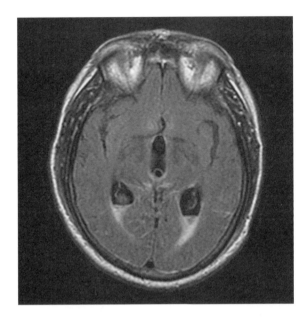

Figure A14.3

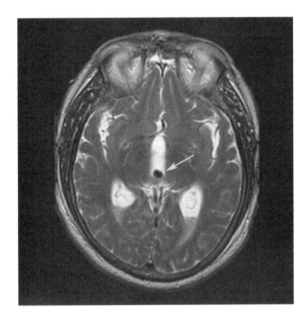

Figure A14.4

While the fluid-fluid levels from hemorrhage in the lateral ventricles are clearly evident on the FLAIR scan (Figure A14.3), it is considerably more difficult to identify the clot in the third ventricle on FLAIR, although it is quite apparent on the T2WI (arrow, Figure A14.4).

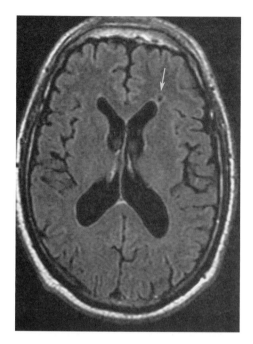

Figure A14.5

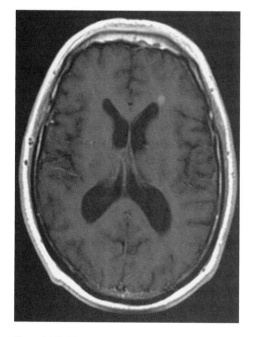

Figure A14.6

The axial FLAIR scan (Figure A14.5) demonstrates what appears to be porencephaly from an old infarct filled with CSF adjacent to the left frontal horn (arrow). This lesion enhances on the T1WI postcontrast scan (Figure A14.6), however, because it is in fact a hemorrhagic metastatic lesion. The susceptibility effect of the hemorrhage caused the signal loss on the FLAIR scan, which, in this case, resembled the expected low-signal appearance of CSF.

Artifact 15

This 50-year-old woman with a history of prior aneurysm surgery and new transient ischemic attacks (TIAs) presents for her MRA. The MIP reconstructions are shown in Figures A15.1 and A15.2. You are concerned that:

(1) she has a high-grade left MCA stenosis.

(2) she has a left MCA occlusion.

(3) You should probably not be reading this MRA without looking at some other imaging.

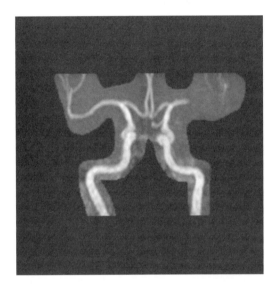

Figure A15.1

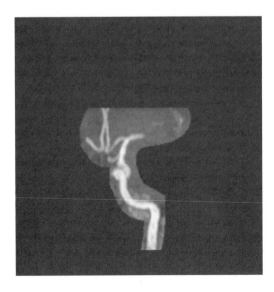

Figure A15.2

SUSCEPTIBILITY ARTIFACTS AND MRA

Yes, this is a difficult question without more imaging. The patient's T2WI image (Figure A15.3) demonstrates a signal void from the aneurysm clip previously placed on her left MCA bifurcation (Figure A15.4). You are probably used to seeing images of patients with aneurysm clips by now, but there was a time when they were scanned with a good deal of trepidation. While clips made from MR-compatible metals like titanium and cobalt alloy have become standard, they still cause large susceptibility artifacts. This is due to the high magnetic permeability of the metal clip compared with the surrounding brain. The susceptibility artifacts from aneurysm clips are sufficient to cause signal loss in the adjacent normal vessel on MRA as well as in the distal vasculature. This is just one reason why it is essential to obtain and review the source images, and ideally at least one T1WI scan, whenever you review an MRA scan (Figures A15.5 and A15.6).

Correct answer: 3

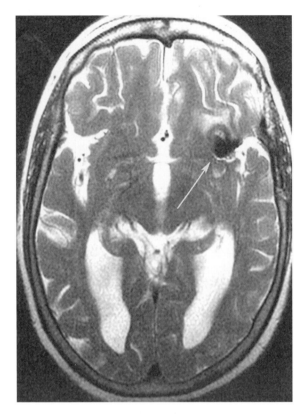

Figure A15.3

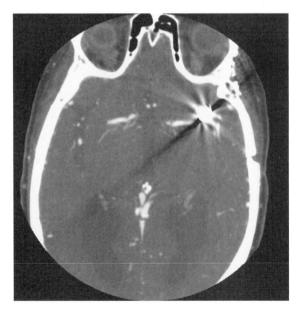

Figure A15.4

The axial T2WI (Figure A15.3) and CT scans (Figure A15.4) show the respective artifacts from this left MCA bifurcation aneurysm clip on MR (Figure A15.3, arrow) and CT.

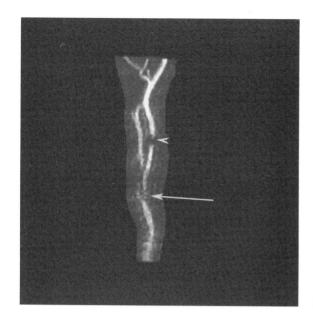

Figure A15.5

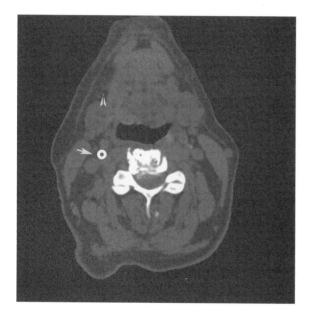

Figure A15.6

This patient presented for his MRA with a history of carotid stenosis. The MIP of the right carotid from his 2D TOF MRA (Figure A15.5) demonstrates what appears to be a proximal stenosis of the internal carotid artery (arrow) as well as a more distal stenosis (arrowhead). This second flow gap turned out to be entirely due to the susceptibility artifact from his right carotid stent, seen here on the CT scan (arrow, Figure A15.6). Follow-up angiography demonstrated that this stent was widely patent.

Artifact 16

This 62-year-old woman presented with worsening headaches and an elevated sedimentation rate. This 3D TOF MRA (Figure A16.1) was obtained to establish the diagnosis of vasculitis. You decide that:

(1) there are multiple stenoses of the left MCA branches.

(2) the patient has an intracranial dissection.

(3) the scan is probably normal.

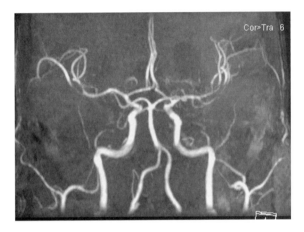

Figure A16.1

3D TOF ARTIFACTS, VENETIAN BLINDS, AND MOTION

This case provides a reminder that MRA of the brain using 3D TOF technique is usually acquired as two to five slabs, unlike the 100 or more thin slices acquired during a 2D TOF sequence. This approach is called MOTSA (multiple overlapping thin slab acquisition). To make 3D TOF images of the intracranial vessels, rather than include all the region of interest in a single slab, multiple thin slabs are acquired with an overlap and then knit together to appear as one continuous volume. The image contrast for both 2D and 3D techniques is still the result of entry slice enhancement, i.e., unsaturated spins coming from outside into an imaged volume, and you may recall that the advantage of 3D TOF imaging in the brain is its improved depiction of curving vessels. These multiple thin slabs are necessary because the hydrogen spins become progressively saturated by the repeated 90 degree pulses as they experience as they traverse the slab. As a result, when using a single, thick slab there would be no signal recovered from the most distal portions of a vessel.

These slabs are acquired sequentially i.e. one after the other. Figure A16.1 demonstrates misregistration between slabs due to some head motion that occurred between two adjacent slab acquisitions. Another common 3D TOF artifact is the loss of flow-related enhancement that becomes increasingly evident as the vessel approaches the exit side of each slab. This phenomenon explains the *Venetian blind artifact* that appears on some 3D TOF images (Figures A16.2 and A16.3) since the intravascular signal varies from bright at the bottom (entry) side to dark at the top. This variation becomes more apparent when the slabs are stitched together.

This signal loss can be corrected, however, by modifying the pulse sequence to "add" vascular signal at the exit side of the slab. This is accomplished by using a variable flip angle on this gradient echo acquisition that changes during each slab acquisition. Since the vascular signal increases with an increase in the flip angle, a modulated or "ramped" flip angle can be used to correct for vascular signal loss. This approach can help to provide a seamless appearance to the vasculature across the multiple slabs (Figure A16.4).

Correct answer: 3

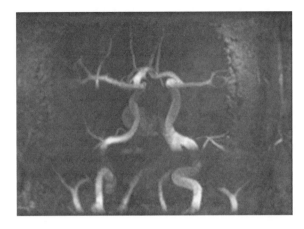

Figure A16.2

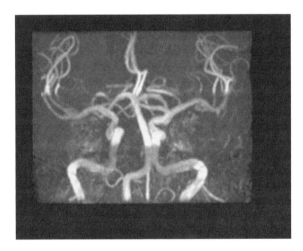

Figure A16.3

These images are examples of Venetian blind artifact due to intravascular signal loss at the exit side of each slab.

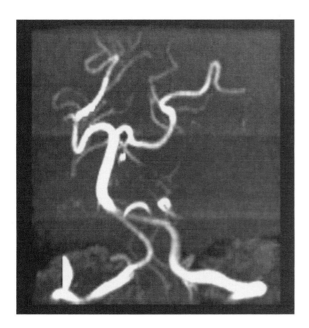

Figure A16.4 This MIP image, created by knitting together three slabs of 3D TOF acquisitions, demonstrates a more uniform signal in the vessels across the three slabs and you can see the change in signal where the slabs overlap.

Artifact 17

This source image from a 3D TOF MRA (Figure A17.1) show a serpiginous high-signal structure in the region of the patient's left temporal lobe. You suspect that this represents:

(1) an AVM.

(2) a large developmental venous anomaly (DVA).

(3) the ear.

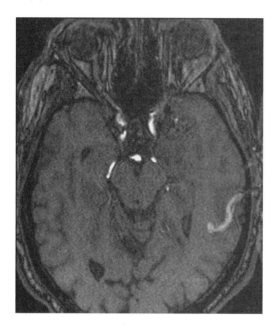

Figure A17.1

WRAPAROUND ARTIFACTS

The axial scout (Figure A17.2) from the patient in A17.1 shows how the right ear, which of course exactly matches the contour of the high signal overlying the temporal lobe, was wrapped into the MRA image. Figures A17.3 and A17.4 illustrate other wraparound artifacts. These occur because spatial location is determined using phase information and since there is some ambiguity with regard to absolute phase shift, i.e., phase shifts of 10 degrees and 370 degrees look about the same to the scanner, the wrong spatial location may be assigned to signal coming from outside the imaging field of view. This artifact usually does not occur in the frequency direction on modern scanners so consider it only in the phase encoding direction. While this is also the direction for flow-related ghosting, that occurs because the protons' phase information is incorrect relative to its actual location. When phase wrap occurs, there is no mistake; it is just that signals from two different spatial locations are assigned to the same place on the image.

There are several ways to minimize this problem. One simple solution is to use a large field of view so that all of the body part is covered within the span of available phase shifts. This approach does not allow for high-resolution imaging with small fields of view, however. Saturation bands or fat suppression can be helpful since they allow you to suppress the signal from tissue outside the image field. To simplify things, it is helpful to intentionally assign the shorter axis of the body to the phase encoding direction since there will simply be less tissue to cover in the available phase steps. Another approach is to *oversample* in the phase direction. This means that the scan is acquired with more phase encoding steps than would seem necessary for the imaged field of view, but the additional phase information is then discarded before image processing, so it doesn't wrap around into the image.

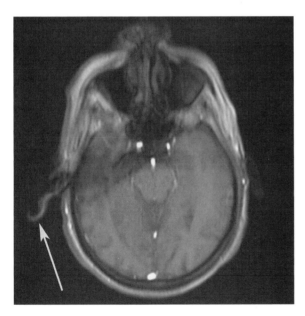

Figure A17.2 This axial scout view reveals that the contour of the right ear (arrow) precisely matches that of the bright structure overlying the left hemisphere. This confirms that the finding on the MRA was only a wraparound artifact, not an abnormal vascular structure.

Correct answer: 3

This artifact is not unique to acquisitions of single slices. Look for its appearance on volume acquisitions in the slice encoding as well as the phase encoding direction. It is important to be aware of this artifact when you interpret images, particularly when using a small field of view, so that the wrapped signal is not mistaken for disease.

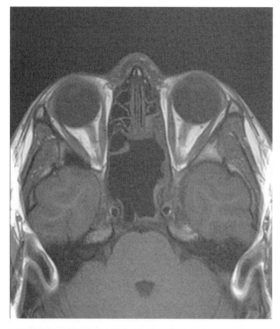

Figure A17.3

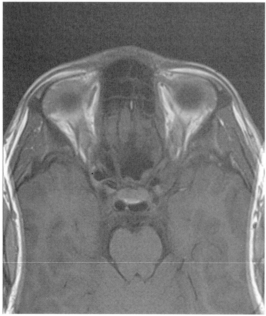

Figure A17.4

These are two other examples of more apparent ear (Figure A17.3) and scalp (Figure A17.4) wraparound artifacts.

Artifact 18

This 54-year-old male with a history of MS was referred for a thoracic cord examination. Linear high signal is evident in the center of the cord on the sagittal T2WI image (Figure A18.1, arrow), but the axial T2WI images at this level are completely normal. You think that this most likely represents:

(1) cord demyelination.

(2) a syrinx.

(3) a Gibbs artifact.

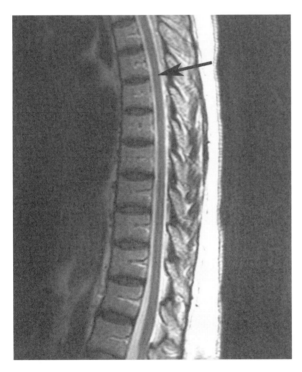

Figure A18.1

TRUNCATION ARTIFACTS

Interpreting thoracic spinal cord MR images can be challenging because artifacts due to pulsations of CSF as well as respiratory motion can project over the spinal cord on T2WI. The artifacts from CSF pulsation can be minimized with the addition of flow compensation techniques, and the nearby fat can be suppressed using STIR or saturation bands. There is, however, one other artifact that can contribute to artifactual high signal in the spinal cord called a *Gibbs artifact*.[1] This is attributed to the difficulties of replicating the sharp changes in contrast between adjacent structures like cord and CSF using limited frequency information. While large data sets will allow a closer approximation of the edge, with limited time and data there will be some "truncation" of the information. This artifact is most evident where there are sharp contrast borders and a coarse matrix is used for the image acquisition. It cannot be entirely eliminated, but it can be minimized by using either a smaller field of view or a larger (finer) matrix. It is not seen often today because fast spin echo imaging and high field scanners has allowed the use of a finer matrix without consuming too much time.

As the matrix increases and the pixels are therefore smaller, this artifact is minimized because the transition at any high-contrast edge is spread over more pixels. In the head, this artifact can be confused with chemical shift (frequency direction) or motion artifact (phase direction), but the Gibbs artifact can usually be differentiated from both since it may be apparent in both directions simultaneously.

Not all bright lines in the spinal cord are due to artifacts, however. The normal gray matter of the cord is usually evident on high-quality MR images of the cervical cord. This can be differentiated from a Gibbs artifact in most cases by location. When the Gibbs artifact is visible, it is located in the exact center of the cord, while the gray matter appears at the junction of the anterior and middle one-third on sagittal imaging. Dilation of the central canal (Figures A18.3 and A18.4) or a small syrinx generally should not be mistaken for a Gibbs artifact. A syrinx tends to be more sharply defined and is evident on both T1WI and T2WI axial imaging.

---

[1] The *s* in *Gibbs* is not the possessive form, like *Occam's razor*; it is part of the discoverer's name. This artifact was named for the American physicist J. Willard Gibbs, who was called "the greatest mind in American history" by Albert Einstein. He became a professor at Yale in 1871, so his work predated NMR by nearly 100 years. There is some irony in attaching his name to this artifact since his life's work focused on the mathematics of what is now called thermodynamics, but the principles of this artifact were described in a brief report. Such are the vagaries of fame.

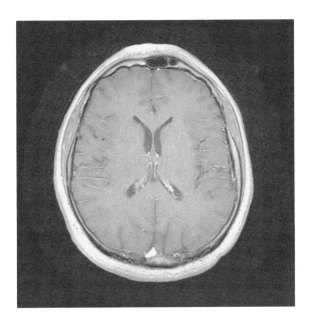

Figure A18.2 Note the "ringing" concentric lines lateral to the right scalp consistent with a Gibbs rtifact.

Correct answer: 3

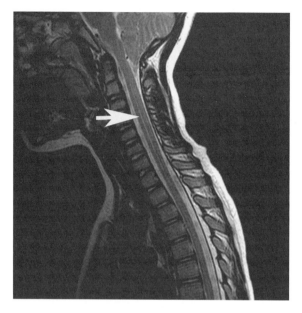

Figure A18.3

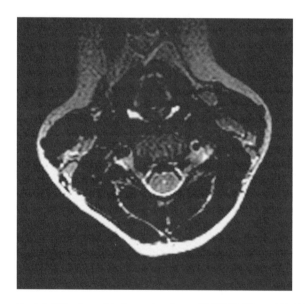

Figure A18.4

The bright line (arrow) in the cord on the sagittal T2WI (Figure A18.3) is due to dilatation of the central canal, not a Gibbs artifact. Note that it is not in the exact center of the cord and is well seen on the axial T2WI as well (Figure A18.4).

Artifact 19

This 45-year-old man presented with ankle pain after playing in his first basketball game since college. His doctor ordered this MR scan (Figures A19.1 and A19.2) with the indication "rule out Achilles tendon rupture." Your see some high signal in the tendon (arrow, Figure A19.1) and decide that it is due to:

(1) an Achilles tendon rupture.

(2) inhomogeneity of the peripheral magnetic field.

(3) a magic angle artifact.

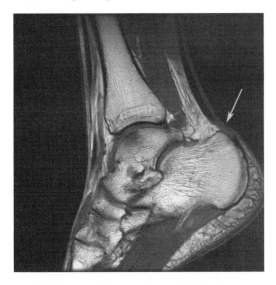

Figure A19.1

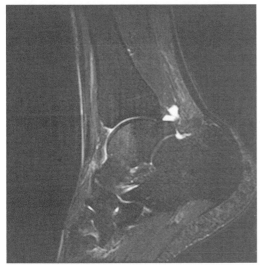

Figure A19.2

(Images provided by Douglas Goodwin, MD, Dartmouth-Hitchcock Medical Center, Lebanon, NH.)

MAGIC ANGLE ARTIFACTS

In highly structured tissues like muscles, we expect to find a relatively short T2 relaxation time due to the ease of spin-spin energy exchange common to any highly structured tissue. Always keep in mind that in water (i.e. CSF) and in lesions with increased interstitial or intracellular water, there will be more opportunities for the hydrogen protons to move about. Their freedom of movement limits their interactions with nearby protons and in part explains the long T1 and T2 relaxation time compared with that of more structured tissues like muscle. One particularly striking example of the effects of structure on T2 relaxation time is the contrast between MR imaging of ice and water (Figure A19.3).

Ice is quite interesting when you consider its transition from liquid water.[2] As water changes into ice, its T1 and T2 relaxation times change as well. T1 relaxation time decreases until, at −35°C, it has decreased by a factor of 10. This shortening of the T1 (spin-lattice) relaxation time reflects the faster transfer of energy from the excited spins of hydrogen in a solid compared with a liquid. But this effect alone cannot explain the loss of signal from ice on a T2-weighted image (Figure A19.3). This is due to the extremely short T2* relaxation time common to all crystalline solids. (Recall that the symbol T2* reflects both the inherent T2 relaxation time of the tissue and the additional signal losses due to inhomogeneities of the magnetic field.) The T2* relaxation time for ice is so short that there is no residual magnetization left in the transverse plane by the time we get around to listening for the returning signal, so it appears black on T2WI. At the same time, the hydrogen nuclei in free water lose phase coherence very slowly because of their limited spin-spin interactions. Therefore, liquid water protons can be brought back to coherent phase with a 180 degree pulse. At the moment of the "echo," the net magnetization arising from voxels that contain water will be sufficiently large to create a strong signal in the antenna, which is then represented as bright signal on the T2-weighted image.

As structure in human tissues goes, tendons represent an extreme. When the fibers of the tendon are oriented along the long axis of the strong magnetic field, the T2 relaxation time of tendons is on the order of *25 microseconds (usec)*. This rapid dephasing of the hydrogen protons bound in the structure of tendons prevents them from contributing recoverable signal. In this dark background, it is easy to see the free water from edema and swelling on MR imaging. In one specific circumstance, however, a portion of a normal tendon may appear to have high signal on MR imaging. This is because the tendon spin-spin interactions also depend on its orientation with respect to the scanner's magnetic field. As the tendon reaches an angle of 55 degrees with the strong magnetic field, its T2 relaxation time increases so much that the tendon may appear bright (Figure A19.1). This phenomenon is called the *magic angle effect*.

---

[2] Ice has another unusual property that proves to be very important for fish and people who live in cold climates. Instead of becoming more compact as it cools, like almost everything else, water becomes most dense just above 0°C, but with any further cooling it expands. In fact, ice is 10% less dense than water. This expansion of ice explains why ice on a lake doesn't sink to the bottom (good for fish). However, it will cause frozen water pipes in your basement to burst (not so good) (Figure 19.4).

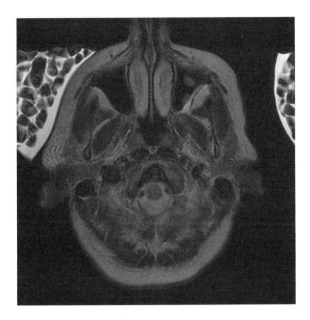

Figure A19.3 This image demonstrates the short T2 relaxation time on T2WI of ice compared with water in this ice bag that was included on this image of a patient with a headache.

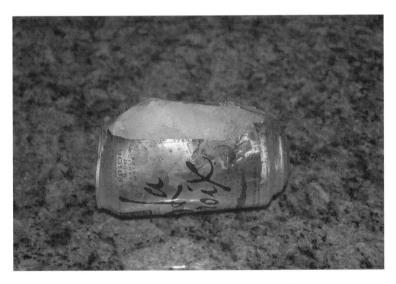

Figure A19.4 This can of water was left outside on a cold night. Notice that it has burst due to the expansion of the ice inside.

Correct answer: 3

You should have been suspicious when the tendon appeared nearly normal on the long TE image (Figure A19.2) since any free water, i.e. edema, should be more evident at longer TE. For example, the free fluid in the joint and the marrow edema in the talus are more conspicuous on this long TE image. Magic angle effects are most apparent on images with short TE times, however, and this is why it is inapparent on Figure A19.2. Because optimal demonstration of musculoskeletal disorders (e.g. meniscal tears) requires TE times in the same range where magic angle effects appear, relying on long TE time pulse sequences to avoid creating this artifact is not an effective strategy. Awareness of this phenomenon should help you to recognize it when it appears, and careful positioning of the joint in the scanner at the time of image acquisition should minimize the magic angle effect from the start.

There really is a bit of magic to it, so if you still need convincing, look at this bovine tendon as it turns from parallel with the main magnetic field into a 55 degree angle (Figures A19.5 and A19.6).

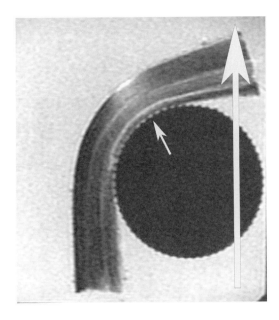

Figure A19.5

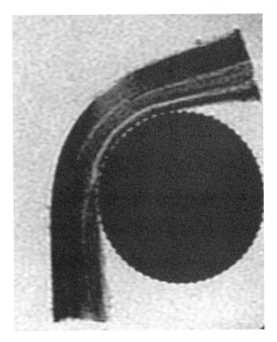

Figure A19.6

Note how the signal within this bovine tendon on a TE 30 msec image (Figure A19.5) increases as it changes from parallel to the axis of the strong magnetic field on your left (0 degrees, large arrow) to an angle of 55 degrees (thin arrow) until it turns to a nearly 90 degree angle with the field at the top of the image. The magic angle effect is much less evident on the TE 60 msec image (Figure A19.6) because it is TE dependent. An understanding of the characteristic appearance of this artifact should help you to distinguish it from true tendon pathology. (Images provided by Douglas Goodwin, MD, Dartmouth-Hitchcock Medical Center, Lebanon, NH.)

Artifact 20

This patient has a history of MS, and this MR scan was obtained to determine if she has active disease. The axial FLAIR scan (Figure A20.1) demonstrates multiple white matter lesions compatible with the diagnosis of MS. The corresponding magnetization transfer T1WI postcontrast scan (Figure A20.2) demonstrates high signal in these same lesions suggesting enhancement that usually indicates active disease. What additional pulse sequence would you need to make this diagnosis with confidence?

    (1) diffusion.

    (2) precontrast T1WI.

    (3) precontrast magnetization transfer.

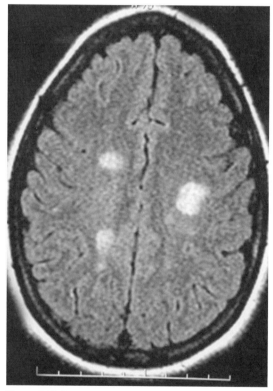

Figure A20.1

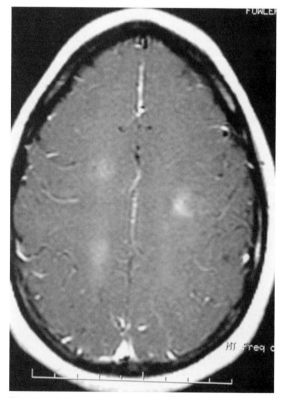

Figure A20.2

MAGNETIZATION SHINE THROUGH ARTIFACT

Magnetization transfer (MT) imaging is another technique, much like chemical fat suppression, that uses a preparatory RF pulse to alter image contrast. Within the brain, there are very large molecules that are invisible on conventional MR images because of their very short T2 relaxation time and, much like dark matter in the cosmos, can only be discerned indirectly by their influence on the hydrogen nuclei that we can image. By applying a preparatory pulse to selectively suppress these large molecules, energy can "transfer" to nearby hydrogen protons and thereby suppress their signal as well. This will have the greatest effect on hydrogen spins in well-structured tissues, while in those regions with less well structured tissue (e.g., MS lesions), hydrogen spins will appear relatively more conspicuous because they will show relatively less suppression. This suppression of normal tissue in order to expose less structured tissue provides yet another source of MR image contrast.

Magnetization transfer contrast has another beneficial effect when used for MR imaging. When used along with contrast enhancement, it offers a relatively inexpensive way to increase the conspicuity of enhancing brain lesions. When imaging the brain, increasing the dose of contrast has the potential to make lesions with no blood-brain barrier, such as metastatic lesions, more evident since the normal brain remains essentially unchanged because it has an intact blood-brain barrier. This additional contrast then increases conspicuity of lesions by exaggerating the lesion-to-background contrast. Magnetization transfer effects can also exaggerate the effect of contrast but in this case the increased conspicuity is due to suppression of the signal from normal brain. The attraction here is that it occurs without the added cost or potential risk of an additional contrast dose.

Unfortunately, in order to discriminate inherent MT tissue contrast from enhancement, it is essential to obtain a precontrast MT scan (Figures A20.3–A20.7). When the two scans are compared in this case, you can see that the lesions on the patients' left (Figure A20.3) are unchanged in appearance from the precontrast MT scan (Figure A20.4). While pure MT imaging is not commonly used because of this additional imaging time and complexity, there are MT effects even on fat-saturated images of the brain that can improve lesion-to-background contrast on postcontrast T1WI.

Correct answer: 3

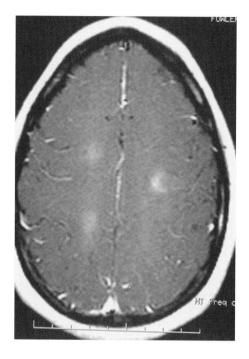

Figure A20.3

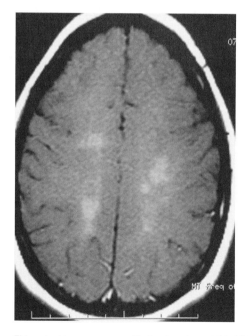

Figure A20.4

This pair of images, a magnetization transfer weighted (MT) noncontrast scan (Figure A20.3) and the same with contrast (Figure A20.4), demonstrate the MT shine-through effect, which can be easily confused with true enhancement unless the precontrast MT scan is also available.

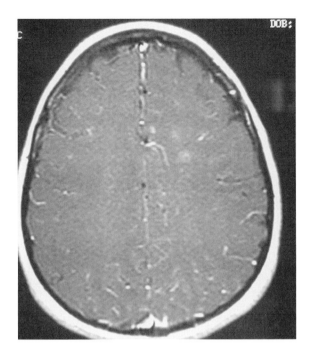

Figure A20.5

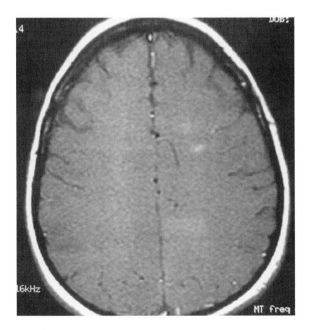

Figure A20.6

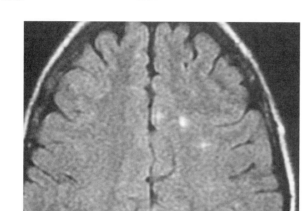

Figure A20.7

This set of images includes a postcontrast MT (Figure A20.5), a precontrast MT (Figure A20.6), and an axial FLAIR (Figure A20.7) scan that provide another example of MT shine through in this patient with MS. This effect should be considered whenever you review postcontrast MT images so that it is not mistaken for evidence of active disease.

Artifact 21

This 25-year-old woman present with severe headaches. You notice that the CSF in the frontal subarachnoid space (Figure A21.1) appears much brighter than that seen in the ventricles or elsewhere in the subarachnoid space. While you should be thinking about meningitis or subarachnoid blood, you are pretty sure that this is:

(1) a susceptibility artifact.

(2) a flow artifact.

(3) a effect of inhaled oxygen.

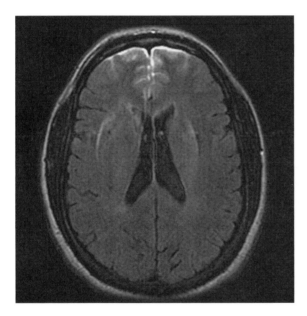

Figure A21.1

PSEUDOSUBARACHNOID HEMORRHAGE ON FLAIR

This case illustrates another manifestation of metal susceptibility artifacts. The very nature of FLAIR imaging depends on precise timing of the 180 and 90 degree pulses. In cases where there is image distortion due to inhomogeneity of the magnetic field, there may be incomplete CSF suppression. Since FLAIR is basically a T2-weighed scan, the CSF will appear bright if it is not successfully suppressed on this pulse sequence. The problem with this particular artifact is that it can easily be mistaken for changes in relaxation of CSF that are usually encountered with hemorrhage or infection.

It is important to view the entire stack of images to determine if there is evidence of metal artifact since these effects may project quite far away from the metal itself. In Figure A21.1, the curvilinear high signal noted on either side of the ventricles is a hint that something is awry. If you had seen this other image from lower in the FLAIR stack (Figure A21.2), the diagnosis would have been easier. FLAIR, much like chemical fat suppression, requires a homogeneous magnetic field to be effective in CSF suppression (Figures A21.3-A21.5).

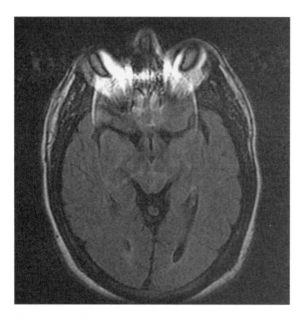

Figure A21.2 This axial FLAIR image at the level of the orbits demonstrates considerable distortion of normal anatomy due to susceptibility artifacts from wire braces.

Correct answer: 1

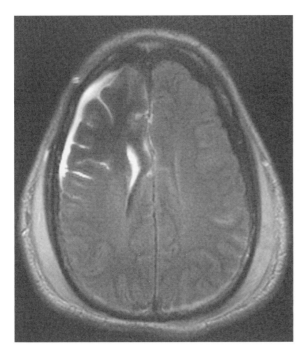

Figure A21.3

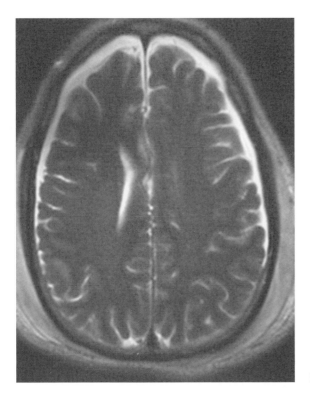

Figure A21.4

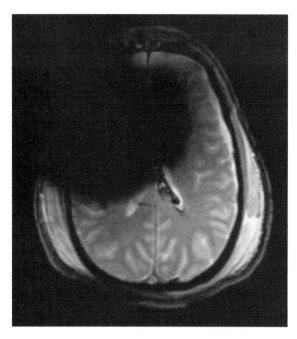

Figure A21.5

The axial FLAIR scan (Figure A21.3) also shows increased signal in the right frontal subarachnoid space, subdural space, and ventricle. While this suggests abnormality of the subarachnoid space, it is entirely due to distortion of the magnetic field from metal artifact. The appearance of the T2WI (Figure A21.4) and the gradient echo scan (Figure A21.5) from the same patient demonstrate the relative sensitivity of these different pulse sequences to this metal artifact. Note the large zone of signal loss on the gradient echo exam compared with the minimal change on the FSE T2 at the same level.

Artifact 22

This coronal gradient echo scan (Figure A22.1), obtained with a TE of 2.2 msec on a 1.5T MR scanner, demonstrates black lines at all the fat–muscle interfaces. You wonder if this is due to:

(1) a susceptibility artifact.

(2) hemosiderosis.

(3) chemical shift.

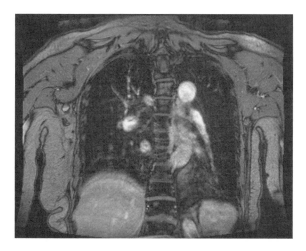

Figure A22.1

CHEMICAL SHIFT CANCELLATION ARTIFACT

The chemical shift cancellation artifact is a variation of the chemical shift artifact (see Artifact 8) and is most evident on gradient echo imaging where TE times are often under 10 msec. Remember that the Larmor frequency for hydrogen protons is proportional to the strength of the magnetic field, but it is also influenced by how the hydrogen atoms are bound. Hydrogen atoms in fat are bound in a large molecule along with carbon, which alters their frequency of precession compared with hydrogen in water by about 4 ppm. Because of the slight difference in their frequencies, the phase of protons in water and fat will drift in and out of phase over time. To picture this, consider the second hand and the hour hand of a wristwatch. If you set the time on an analog watch using the winder stem, you will see the minute hand spin around rapidly while the hour hand moves more slowly. This is because they are spinning at different frequencies, just like protons in water and fat. At 1:05, when the second hand covers the hour hand, they could be described as *in phase*. At 12:30, however, when they point in opposite directions, they could be described as *out of phase*. When the hydrogen protons of both fat and water are in phase, their magnetic fields add together to increase their net magnetization. However, when they are out of phase, their net magnetization cancel because they point in opposite directions; this effect is called *chemical shift cancellation*. At a magnetic field of 1.5 T, protons in water and fat will be in phase at a TE of 4.4 msec and out of phase at a TE of 2.2 msec.

This phenomenon can be used to advantage when doing MRA where suppression of fat is helpful in order to prevent visualization of short T1 tissues. In some circumstances, i.e. an intracranial lipoma, the high signal of fat (short T1 relaxation) can be mistaken for the high signal of flow (flow related enhancement) since both will appear on the TOF images. The unwanted visualization of fat or blood on TOF imaging is also called "shine through". The fat signal can be minimized on a 3D TOF scan by choosing a TE where fat and water protons cancel. This technique is also used for diagnostic imaging to characterize any fat-containing mass. For example, the presence of fat in an adrenal mass can help to establish the diagnosis of a benign adenoma based on the change in signal of the mass on TE 2.2 and 4.4 images (Figures A22.2 and A22.3).

Where both fat and water appear in the same voxel, which should be expected at fat–tissue interfaces, phase cancellation will make those voxels appear black. This will be visible on imaging as circumferential black lines around muscles, much like the way a cartoon is drawn. This can be easily discriminated from the dark line visible with the usual chemical shift artifact that is evident at longer TE times since that artifact is only visible in the frequency direction.

Correct answer: 3

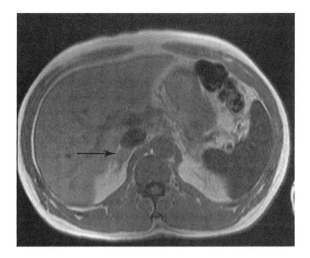

Figure A22.2

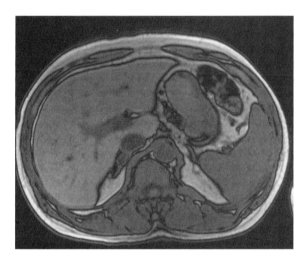

Figure A22.3

These axial abdominal images were obtained using a TE of 4.4 and 2.2. The adrenal mass seen on the TE 4.4 image (Figure A22.2, arrow) shows a sharp drop in signal on the TE 2.2 image (Figure A22.3). This is due to phase shift cancellation effects from the out-of-phase hydrogen protons in water and fat intermixed within this benign adrenal adenoma. Note the dark appearance of the margin of the liver and spleen on this TE 2.2 msec image as well. This is another example of a chemical shift cancellation artifact.

Artifact 23

This 80-year-old patient presents with symptoms of TIA. An MRA scan of the neck was requested.

These MIP images of the left (Figure A23.1) and right (Figure A23.2) carotid circulations were created from the 2D TOF data set. Note the apparent narrowing in both carotids at the skull base (arrows). Your diagnosis?

(1) bilateral spontaneous carotid dissections.

(2) turbulent flow artifacts.

(3) susceptibility artifacts.

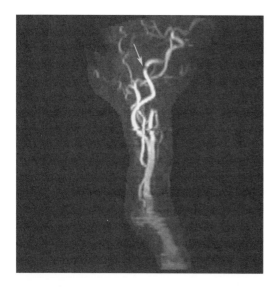

Figure A23.1

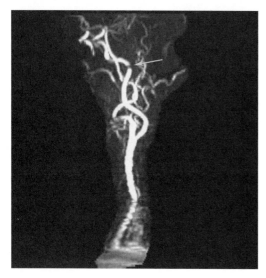

Figure A23.2

2D TOF SUSCEPTIBILITY ARTIFACTS

Two-dimensional TOF imaging is acquired as multiple slices using a gradient echo technique. Since the source images are acquired individually, it is common to encounter movement on one or more slices that will appear shifted in the stack on MIP reconstructions like coins out of line in a stack (Figures A23.3 and A23.4). While motion is certainly a plausible explanation for the focal narrowing evident in both carotids in this case, the narrowing cannot be attributed to patient motion because it is not seen in any branches of the external carotid arteries, and misregistration alone would be evident in those vessels as well.

The patient went on to have a gadolinium arch MRA scan that demonstrated an entirely normal contour of the carotids (Figure A23.5). This artifactual narrowing of the carotids at the skull base reflects the susceptibility effects, with associated signal loss in the vessels, at the interface of soft tissue and bone at the skull base. This would explain why the external carotids are normal since, with the exception of the middle meningeal artery, those branches are extracranial.

Correct answer: 3

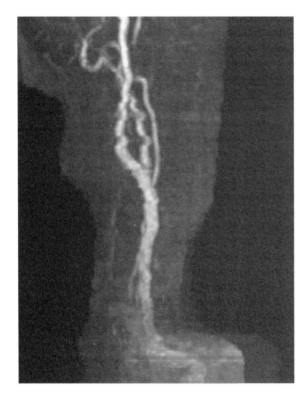

Figure A23.3

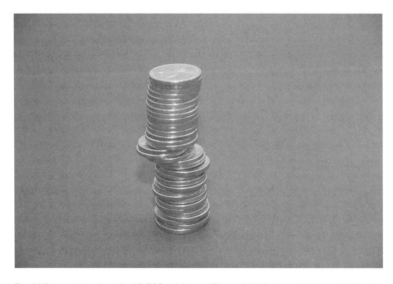

Figure A23.4

The MIP reconstruction of a 2D TOF axial scan (Figure A23.3) shows the irregular border of the carotid due to patient motion, usually from swallowing, during the acquisition. The stack of nickels (Figure A23.4) illustrates how this effect of motion, during acquisition of a few slices of the 2D TOF stack, will create an irregular vascular margin on a reconstructed MIP image.

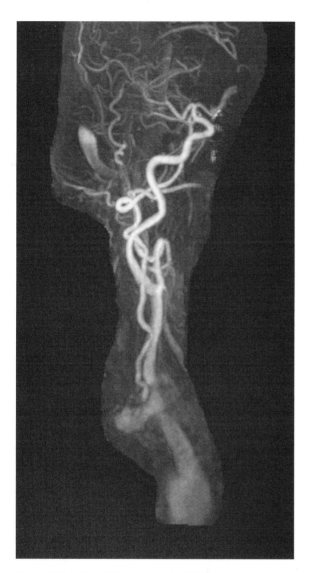

Figure A23.5 The MIP from the contrast MRA shows a normal appearance of the internal carotid with no evidence of narrowing at the skull base.

Artifact 24

The sagittal T1WI (Figure A24.1) demonstrates a high-signal Rathke's cyst in the posterior sella (arrow). This intra-sellar lesion on the same T1WI scan but after the administration of gadolinium contrast (Figure A24.2) now appears dark. This is due to:

(1) fat suppression.

(2) susceptibility effects in the cyst.

(3) windowing.

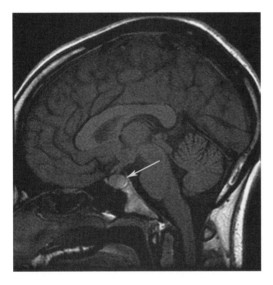

Figure A24.1

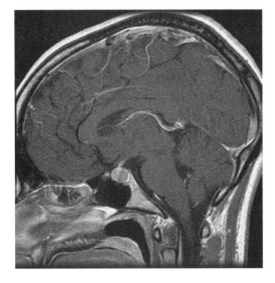

Figure A24.2

IMAGE SCALING ARTIFACTS

The *scaling* effect is more of an illusion than an artifact. It is not reasonable to think that the lesion in the pituitary, which we know was bright on the same scan sequence just before administration of contrast, would suddenly become darker. It appears relatively dark, however, because the adjacent pituitary now appears brighter by comparison with the Rathke's cyst. It cannot be attributed to fat suppression because you can see the fat in the subcutaneous space, so no fat suppression was used on this exam. While susceptibility effects may well play a role in the appearance of Rathke's cysts on T2WI (Figures A24.3 and A24.4), on T1WI susceptibility generally has little impact on image contrast.

Correct answer: 3

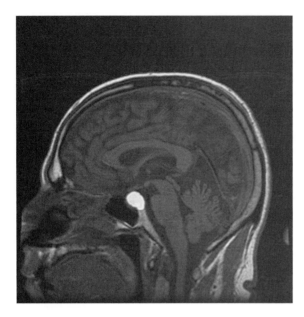

Figure A24.3

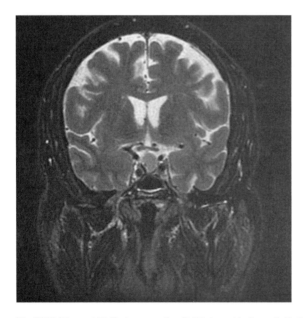

Figure A24.4

The T1WI (Figure A24.3) shows another Rathke's cyst in the sella that is very bright on T1WI but appears dark on T2WI (Figure A24.4). This pattern is typical for a proteinaceous cyst, where the blood products and the high protein provide T1 shortening as well as T2 shortening, making it appear relatively dark on T2WI.

Artifact 25

This T1WI of the abdomen of a child in the newborn nursery (Figure A25.1) shows an air-fluid level in the stomach with very bright gastric contents. This is due to:

(1) something the child ate.

(2) bleeding into the stomach.

(3) field inhomogeneity effects.

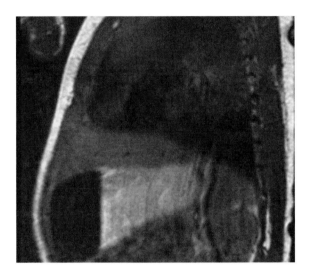

Figure A25.1

T1 EFFECTS OF FORMULA AND PARAMAGNETIC CONTRAST

The appearance of this stomach can be attributed to a recent feeding with formula. The T1 shortening evident in the stomach and bowel lumen on MR images due to formula is so striking that formula has been advocated for use as a diagnostic gastrointestinal contrast agent. The T1 shortening does not appear to be due to fat content in the formula since breast milk, also with a high fat content, does not have the same effect. This T1 shortening is most likely due to dissolved elements like manganese in the formula that are added as nutritional supplements.

Manganese, in particular, is a powerful paramagnetic contrast agent and behaves much like gadolinium on MR. That is because they both have many unpaired electrons, which gives them some paramagnetic properties.

Contrast agents used for X-ray imaging are visible because they attenuate X-rays more than adjacent soft tissues. Magnetic resonance contrast agents, however, are seen only indirectly by their influence on nearby protons' T1 and T2 relaxation times. T1 relaxation time is a measure of the time it takes the energized protons to return to their baseline state of energy, and the speed of this relaxation reflects in some ways how the protons are bound. Just as T2 relaxation time can be predicted by considering the degree of structure of the hydrogen spins (see Artifact 19), T1 relaxation time can be predicted in part by the size of the molecule to which the protons are attached. Larger molecules, like fat, tend to have shorter T1 relaxation times than small molecules, like water. This is attributed to better matching of the frequency of the tumbling rate of these large molecules to the Larmor frequency, which leads to a faster rate of energy dispersal from small fluctuations in the local magnetic field.

When hydrogen spins in water are in the vicinity of a paramagnetic contrast agent like gadolinium, they interact with the contrast agent. Since the contrast augments the local magnetic field this interaction facilitates their T1 relaxation. Because the protons in the vicinity of the gadolinium now have shorter T1 relaxation times, the whole neighborhood where the contrast molecule resides will appear bright on T1WI.

This effect of paramagnetic ions helps to explain why tap water appears very different on MR imaging than distilled water. If you try to test FLAIR techniques with a phantom, for example, you will quickly find that tap water does not suppress at the same TI time as CSF or distilled water. This is because the metal ions in tap water shorten its T1 relaxation time sufficiently for the water protons to recover well past the zero point when the 90 degree pulse is applied. Let's hope they are good for you too.

This effect of manganese in particular is the best explanation for the high signal intensity on T1WI that is evident in the globus pallidus in patients with cirrhosis or on total parenteral nutrition (TPN). The liver regulates how much manganese gets to the body from the ingested food by dumping any excess into the bile which is then excreted back into the gut. Brewer's yeast and coffee are high in manganese, for example, and might otherwise raise serum levels. In the case of cirrhosis, however, the portal blood returning from the gut can bypass the liver via varices and as a reusult the serum manganese levels can rise. With IV TPN, everything bypasses the portal system, of course, and so

Correct answer: 1

again the liver cannot regulate the serum manganese level. When there is an elevated serum manganese level there seems to be active transport of the manganese into the brain, preferentially to the globus pallidus, where it shortens the T1 relaxation time (Figures A25.2 and A25.3). It is of considerable interest that this effect can be reversed in cirrotic patients after liver transplants and may play a role in movement disorders in some patients.

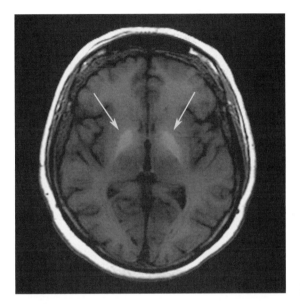

Figure A25.2

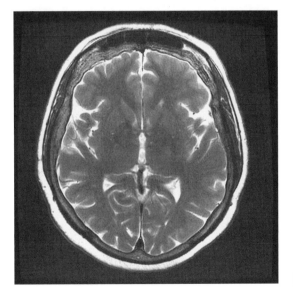

Figure A25.3

The axial T1WI (Figure A25.2) in this patient with cirrhosis demonstrates high signal in the globus pallidus (arrows) due to the effects of manganese, a paramagnetic element. Note that on the T2WI (Figure A25.3) the basal ganglia appear completely normal since the concentration of manganese is so low that only the T1 effects are evident.

Artifact 26

This patient presented with a palpable thigh mass. The axial T1WI (Figure A26.1) demonstrates a rounded soft tissue tumor extending nearly to the skin. The postcontrast scan was obtained using chemical fat suppression (Figure A26.2). The tumor, a sarcoma, has inhomgeneous enhancement, but there is now a low-signal band laterally (arrow). This is due to:

(1) incomplete fat suppression.

(2) T2* shortening from high contrast concentration.

(3) water suppression.

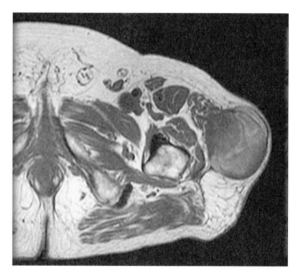

Figure A26.1 (Image provided by Douglas Goodwin, MD, Dartmouth-Hitchcock Medical Center, Lebanon, NH.)

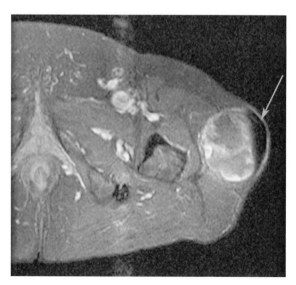

Figure A26.2 (Image provided by Douglas Goodwin, MD, Dartmouth-Hitchcock Medical Center, Lebanon, NH.)

INADVERTENT WATER SUPPRESSION

Chemical fat suppression is based on the principle that the Larmor frequency of hydrogen bound in fat differs from that of hydrogen bound in water. If a 90 degree RF pulse is tuned to the precise frequency of fat, then only fat-bound hydrogen spins will resonate. This technique, however, presumes a homogeneous magnetic field within the scanner. The magnetic field of any MR scanner is most homogeneous in the center, with more irregularity at the periphery.

Occasionally, this inhomogeneity of the magnetic field creates a situation where the Larmor frequency of water varies to the point that it now matches that of fat elsewhere in the scanner. Remember that the Larmor frequency is proportional to the magnetic field, and the inherent difference between fat and water is less than 4 ppm. In this circumstance, the RF pulse used to suppress fat in one place can suppress the signal from hydrogen protons elsewhere. This artifact is usually seen only in body and musculoskeletal MR imaging since nearly all neuroimaging occurs near the midline of the scanner, where the field is more homogeneous (Figures A26.3 and A26.4).

Correct answer: 3

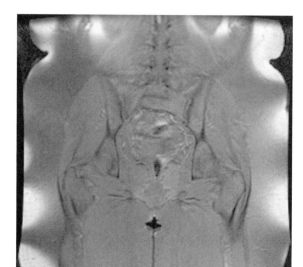

Figure A26.3

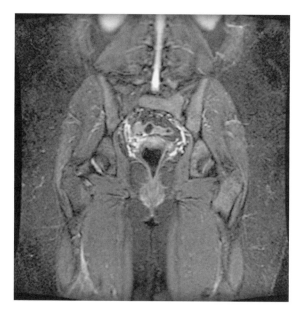

Figure A26.4

Figure A26.3 was obtained using chemical fat suppression. Note how the inhomogeneity of the magnet field at the periphery of the scanner bore leads to incomplete fat suppression of the subcutaneous fat in the lateral thighs and hips. Figure A26.4, of the same patient during the same exam, shows homogeneous fat suppression using a STIR scan because that technique is much less sensitive to small variations in the field. (Image provided by Douglas Goodwin, MD, Dartmouth-Hitchcock Medical Center, Lebanon, NH.)

Artifact 27

This 20-year-old female presents with new headaches. Her doctor ordered an MR scan of the brain. This 5 mm sagittal T1WI (Figure A27.1, left) revealed a well-defined area of low signal in the sella (arrow). The coronal contrast scan, however, was normal (Figure A27.1, right). You are suspicious and call the patient's doctor but find that she has no symptoms or laboratory abnormalities to suggest a pituitary tumor. Your explanation for this finding is:

(1) flow-related ghosting.

(2) a nonfunctioning microadenoma.

(3) a partial volume artifact.

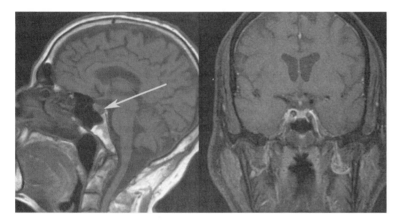

Figure A27.1

PARTIAL VOLUME ARTIFACTS

Partial volume artifacts are commonplace on both MR and CT. Because the signal from a voxel is the composite of all the information within, abnormal tissue can be obscured due to averaging with surrounding normal tissue (Figure A27.2). That is why thin section imaging is so helpful for defining small tumors like microadenomas. With thicker sections, different but normal adjacent structures can also appear on the slice with the pituitary. On Figure A27.1 the flow void from the carotid appeared to be within the pituitary. Thin sagittal imaging (3 mm instead of 5 mm) of the pituitary confirmed that the pituitary was normal (Figure A27.3).

With MR, as slice thickness decreases, the signal from each voxel decreases since there are fewer hydrogen nuclei to contribute to the net magnetization. Let's examine how this may appear in practice. Figure A27.4 is thinner than Figure A27.5 but otherwise the pulse sequences are identical. While you might expect small MS lesions to be more evident on the thinner sections, since there should be less volume averaging, notice that the periventricular white matter lesions are more apparent in Figure A27.5. That is because in order to take full advantage of thinner sections, the pulse sequence needs to be modified to offset signal loss since there are now fewer hydrogen nuclei in each voxel. This predictable signal loss can be offsest by increasing the number of scan acquisitions or decreasing the TE.

Correct answer: 3

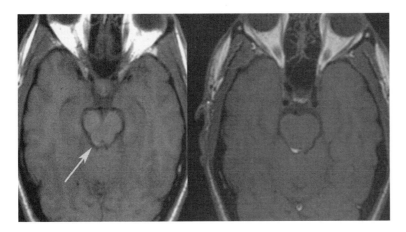

Figure A27.2 The axial 5 mm T1WI (left) shows only subtle high signal in the posterior midbrain (arrow). The 3 mm section at the same level better demonstrates this quadrageminal cistern lipoma because the high signal is not averaged with the normal brain and CSF in these smaller voxels.

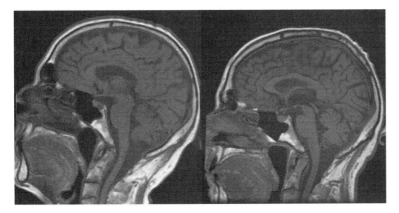

Figure A27.3 The 5 mm sagittal T1WI (Figure A27.1) is on the left and the 3 mm sagittal midline scan (Figure A27.2) is on the right. Note that the pituitary gland appears completely normal on the thinner section.

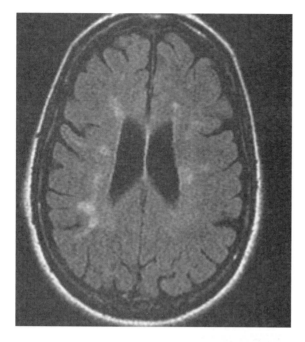

Figure A27.4

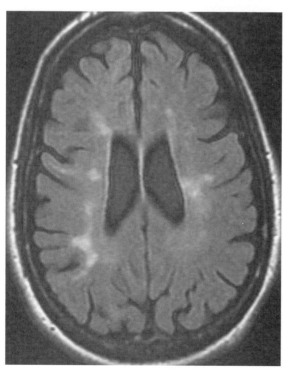

Figure A27.5

This pair of images at the same level were obtained with slice thickness of 3mm (A27.4) and 5mm (A27.5) with all other parameters the same. Notice the poor image quality of 27.4 which is from low signal to noise since there are fewer hydrogen spins available for imaging in these smaller voxels.

Suggested Readings

Byder M, Rahal A, Fullerton GD. The magic angle effect: a source of artifact, determinant of image contrast, and technique for imaging. *J Magn Reson Imaging.* 2007;25:290–300.

Czervionke LF, Czervionke JM, Daniels DL, et al. Characteristic features of MR truncation artifacts. *AJR.* 1988;151:1219–1228.

Davis WL, Blatter DD, Harnsberger R, et al. Intracranial MR angiography: comparison of single-volume three-dimensional time-of-flight and multiple overlapping thin slab acquisition techniques. *AJR.* 1994;163:915–920.

Gerscovich EO, McGahan JP, Buonocore MH, et al. The rediscovery of infant feeding formula with magnetic resonance imaging. *Pediatr Radiol.* 1990;20:147–151.

Haacke EM, Mittal S, Wu Z, et al. Susceptibility-weighted imaging: technical aspects and clinical applications, Part 1. *AJNR.* 2009;30:19–30.

Hajnal JV, Oatridge A, Herlihy AH, et al. Reduction of CSF artifacts on FLAIR images by using adiabatic inversion pulses. *AJNR.* 2001;22:317–322.

Kallmes DF, Hui FK, Mugler JP. Suppression of cerebrospinal fluid and blood flow artifacts in FLAIR MR imaging with a single-slab three-dimensional pulse sequence: initial experience. *Radiology.* 2001;221:251–255.

Knauth M, Forsting M, Hartmann M, et al. MR enhancement of brain lesions: increased contrast dose compared with magnetization transfer. *AJNR.* 1996;17:1853–1859.

Peh WCG, Chan JHM. The magic angle phenomenon in tendons: effect of varying the MR echo time. *Br J Radiol.* 1998;71:31–36.

Shuman WP, Lambert DT, Patten RM, et al. Improved fat suppression in STIR MR imaging: selecting inversion time through spectral display. *Radiology.* 1991;178:885–887.

Wolf SD, Balaban RS. Magnetization transfer imaging: practical aspects and clinical applications. *Radiology.* 1994;192:593–599.

3 MR PITFALLS

In the process of selecting these cases, it occurred to me that one could argue about the classification of some of them as an artifact or a pitfall. Guy Del Villano, who ran a fire equipment company in my hometown and gave me my first real job, forgave my errors but would retell this story about ones that I should have anticipated: "You walkin along, you seea da hole, you fall in, you breaka your leg, at'sa no bad luck, dat's dumb." The intent of these cases is to point out to you some of the holes you may encounter along the way.

Pitfall 1

This 17-year-old young man with a history of head trauma and syncope had a cervical MRA scan. This axial source image from his 2D TOF (Figure P1.1), at the level of the proximal internal carotid, and the reconstructed MIP (Figure P1.2) demonstrate low signal in the posterior bulb (arrow in Figure P1.2). Do you think this is due to:

(1) early atherosclerosis, perhaps the result of eating too much junk food during high school?

(2) reversed flow?

(3) intravoxel dephasing?

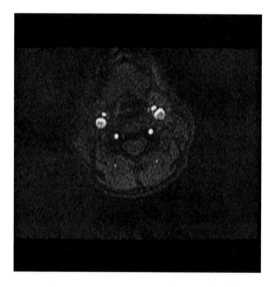

Figure P1.1

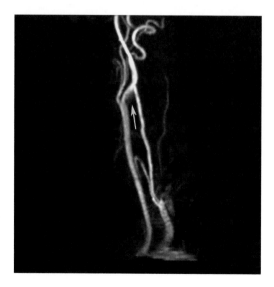

Figure P1.2

RECIRCULATION FLOW ARTIFACTS ON 2D TOF

In young patients with vigorous flow and normal expansion in the proximal internal carotid, called the *carotid bulb*, there is in fact a normal eddy circulation with reversed flow within the bulb. This reversed flow leads to diminished signal on 2D TOF MRA because of the linked saturation band that suppresses all caudal flow, regardless of its nature. The contrast exam, which is insensitive to direction of flow, demonstrates the normal contour of the carotid bulb (Figures P1.3-P1.5).

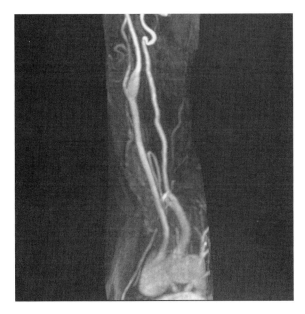

Figure P1.3 The reconstructed contrast enhanced 3D MRA of the same patient demonstrates a normal appearance of the carotid bulb in the same projection as Figure P1.2.

Correct answer: 2

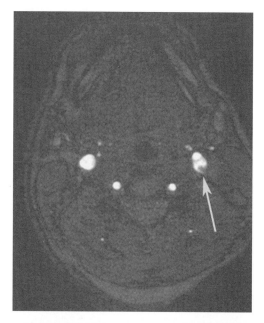

Figure P1.4

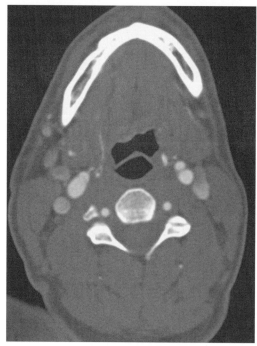

Figure P1.5

This axial image (Figure P1.4) from a cervical 2D TOF MRA of a patient with a history of acute left hemispheric stroke shows low signal in the left proximal internal carotid (arrow). This finding suggests stenosis from atherosclerotic disease. The patient also had a CTA, however, which demonstrated a perfectly normal vessel lumen (Figure P1.5) at the same level. This is another example of how flow suppression of the eddy flow in a normal carotid bulb on 2D TOF can mimic atherosclerotic disease.

Pitfall 2

There is a signal void near the left orbital apex (Figure P2.1, arrow). You think this is due to:

(1) a flow void from a para-ophthlamic aneurysm.

(2) a susceptibility artifact from an aneurysm clip.

(3) air.

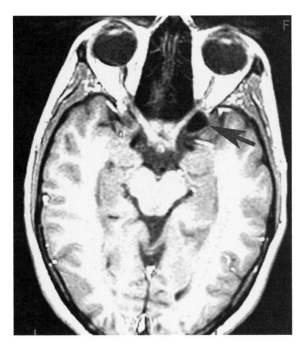

Figure P2.1

PNEUMATIZED ANTERIOR CLINOID

Figure P2.1 illustrates a typical pneumatized anterior clinoid. This is a very common imaging pitfall since clinoids are frequently asymmetrically pneumatized, and the signal void due to low proton density may be mistaken for a flow void from an aneurysm (see Artifact 10). The absence of any flow-related artifact in the phase direction argues against an aneurysm, however. Figure P2.2, the coronal T1WI, provides even more convincing evidence of an air-filled clinoid.

Figure P2.3 shows a pneumatized clinoid in a different patient who had an MRA for left-sided parenchymal hemorrhage (Figure P2.4). You can usually make this diagnosis without any additional imaging, but in some cases it is reassuring to obtain a limited CT scan without contrast to confirm the benign nature of this finding (Figure P2.5).

A reasonable concern is whether one can reliably distinguish a pneumatized anterior clinoid from an aneurysm in all cases. At the outset, it is worthwhile to recognize that an asymmetric pneumatized anterior clinoid is a common finding; therefore, the prior probability favors that diagnosis. However, in all cases, you must look for specific imaging features to support that diagnosis. Since this signal void is entirely due to low proton density (bone and air), you may see susceptibility artifacts but you should never see any motion artifacts (Figures P2.6 and P2.7).

In this location, the presence of flow artifacts, particularly on the contrast scan, argues strongly for moving blood in an aneurysm (Figures P2.8–P2.11). It is helpful to window the image so that you can look into the dark background for these motion artifacts in the phase direction. You can always check to see if the patient had a previous CT or CTA scan; if so, a pneumatized anterior clinoid will be apparent. Finally, the signal void should conform precisely to the expected location of the anterior clinoid. If you have any uncertainty about this diagnosis, consider follow-up with CT, CTA or MRA depending on your level of suspicion.

Correct answer: 3

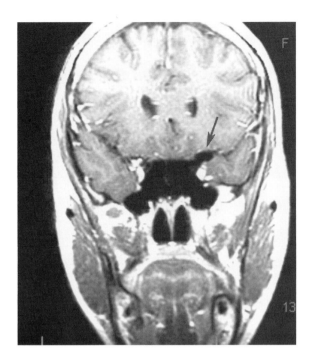

Figure P2.2 This coronal T1WI postcontrast scan shows low signal in the left anterior clinoid (arrow) with no flow ghosting artifacts due to low proton density, i.e., air.

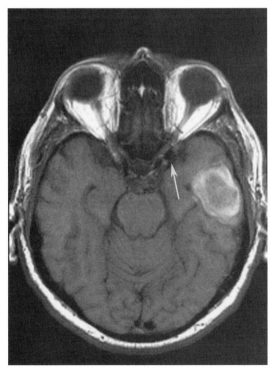

Figure P2.3

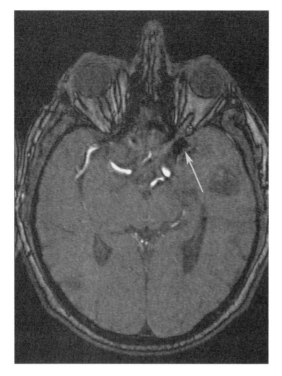

Figure P2.4

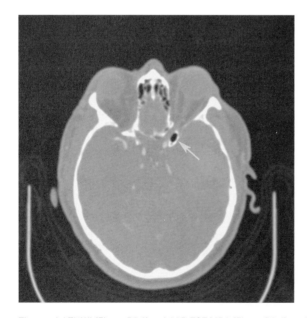

Figure P2.5

These axial TI1WI (Figure P2.3), axial 3D TOF MRA (Figure P2.4), and CTA (Figure P2.5) scans all demonstrate a left-sided pneumatized anterior clinoid (arrows).

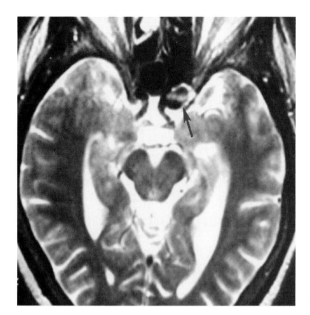

Figure P2.6

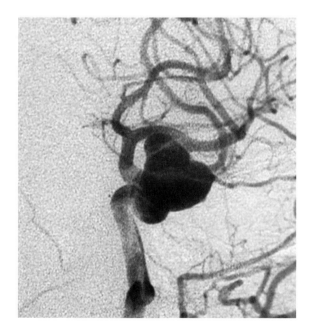

Figure P2.7

This axial T2WI (Figure P2.6) at first glance suggests a pneumatized anterior clinoid on the left (arrow). Note, however, that there is a band of high signal within the signal void suggesting flow. This image from a conventional angiogram (Figure P2.7) confirms the presence of a large carotid aneurysm, which accounts for the inhomogeneous signal evident on Figure P2.6.

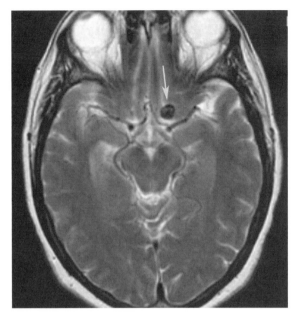

Figure P2.8

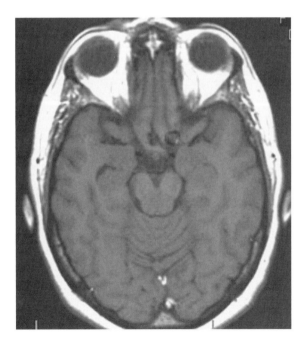

Figure P2.9

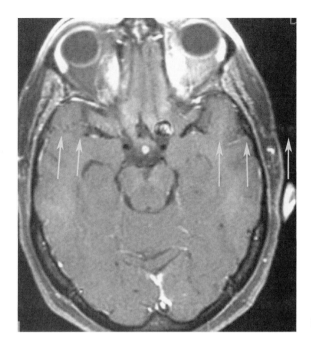

Figure P2.10

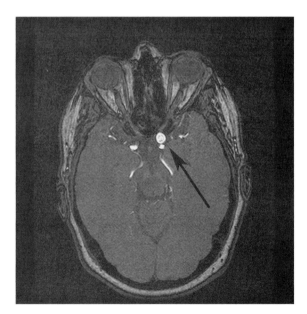

Figure P2.11

The axial T2WI (Figure P2.8) in this 45-year-old woman reveals a signal void near the orbital apex (arrow), but it appears above the level where you might expect to see a pneumatized anterior clinoid. The axial T1WI (Figure P2.9) demonstrates some central high signal and phase artifacts on the postcontrast T1WI (Figure P2.10, arrows) indicating flow. This paraophthalmic aneurysm was confirmed on the 3D TOF MRA (Figure P2.11, arrow).

Pitfall 3

This 50-year-old male developed acute back pain with lower extremity weakness. This MR scan, which was obtained urgently, demonstrates on the T1WI (Figure P3.1) a mass in the dorsal thoracic canal with T1 shortening (arrow). That high signal was suppressed completely, along with the sub-cutaneous and paraspinal fat on the STIR image (Figure P3.2). Based on the symptoms and imaging, you think this is an:

(1) intraspinal lipoma.

(2) epidural abscess.

(3) epidural hemorrhage.

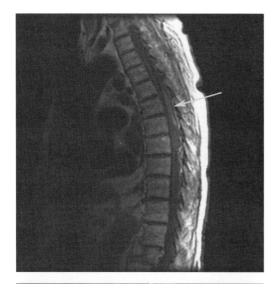

Figure P3.1

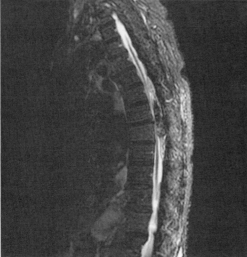

Figure P3.2

STIR PITFALLS

Not all image elements that appear dark on STIR imaging are fat. STIR is usually a T2 weighted inversion recovery sequence that uses a short TI interval in order to suppress tissues with short T1 relaxation times such as fat. However, blood, fat, and gadolinium contrast may all have comparable short T1 relaxation times that are in the T1 range that will be suppressed by STIR. The pitfall in this case is to assume that since the fat is suppressed, all tissue that was bright on the T1WI and dark on STIR is also fat. On the axial T2 scan (Figure P3.3) you can see that the intraspinal mass remains dark, while the subcutaneous fat now appears bright. That indicates that the low signal of the hemorrhage both on T2WI, and the STIR image (Figure P3.2) is due to the susceptibility effects of this acute hemorrhage. So keep in mind that there are several reasons why high signal on T1WI may be suppressed on STIR imaging (Figures P3.4 and P3.5). This case should serve as a reminder that you need to be sure that your diagnosis explains the findings on all the pulse sequences because there may be several reasons why a lesion may appear dark or bright on any one sequence.

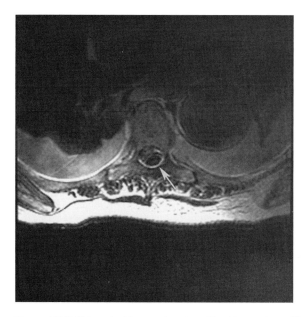

Figure P3.3 This patient has a subacute epidural hemorrhage. The short T1 relaxation time of this hemorrhage was apparent on the T1WI, but the low signal on STIR could be due to either suppression of short T1 tissues or T2* effects. This T2WI shows that signal loss in the region of the dorsal mass consistent with T2* effects (arrow).

Correct answer: 3

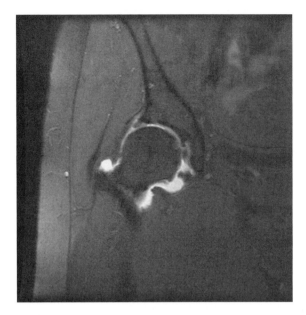

Figure P3.4

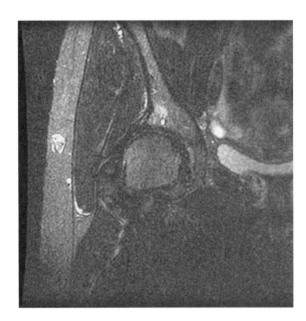

Figure P3.5

This coronal T1WI (Figure P3.4) was obtained using chemical fat suppression and nicely demonstrates the intra-articular gadolinium contrast that had been injected into the right hip joint. Figure P3.5 is a STIR sequence obtained immediately afterward that demonstrates not only suppression of fat signal but also the contrast in the joint space (note the bright signal from the bladder on this T2-weighted image). This is because both the contrast enhanced joint fluid and the fat have similar short T1 relaxation times and STIR imaging does not allow discrimination of one from the other. (Images provided by Douglas Goodwin, MD, Dartmouth-Hitchcock Medical Center, Lebanon, NH.)

Pitfall 4

This 67-year-old male presents with a sudden change in hearing. His exam was consistent with a sensorineural hearing loss in the right ear, and an MR scan with contrast was ordered. This revealed high signal in the right petrous bone (Figures P4.1 and P4.2). What is your diagnosis?

(1) normal.

(2) a vestibular schwannoma.

(3) a CPA meningioma.

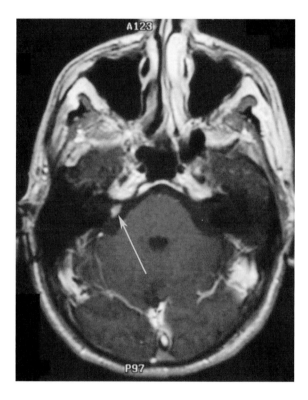

Figure P4.1

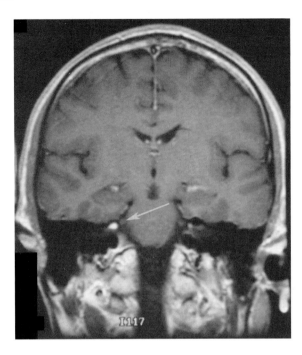

Figure P4.2

VOLUME AVERAGING WITH BONE MARROW

The petrous apex, like the anterior clinoid, is frequently asymmetric. This creates some confusion on MR imaging of the posterior fossa. The axial scan in this patient shows a tongue of fat extending above the internal auditory canal (IAC) (Figure P4.3) that could be easily mistaken for enhancement on a contrast enhanced T1WI when it is performed without fat suppression. The key to making the correct diagnosis in this case is that the normal IAC, where vestibular schwannomas will occur, does not abut the inferior temporal lobe as in Figure P4.2 but lies more caudal in the temporal bone.

Chemical fat suppression can be very helpful for MR contrast examinations of the IAC if used on at least one plane of imaging (Figure P4.4). Keep in mind, however, that you should acquire at least one precontrast thin section T1WI of the IAC in order to make the diagnosis of the rare IAC lipoma (Figures P4.5 and P4.6), which may be symptomatic. An IAC lipoma may prove to be inconspicuous on FIESTA imaging as well (Figure P4.7).

Correct answer: 1

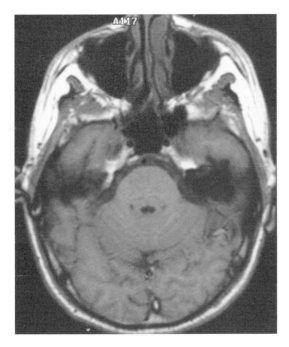

Figure P4.3 This axial T1 scan, which is slightly cephalad to Figure P4.1, better demonstrates the prominent marrow fat . This may be averaged with the IAC on axial sections and therefore resemble abnormal enhancement on T1WI postcontrast imaging unless chemical fat suppression is utilized.

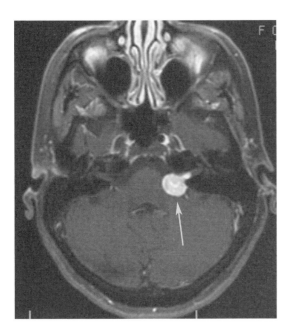

Figure P4.4 This axial fat-suppressed T1WI with contrast demonstrates an enhancing mass in the CPA and IAC (arrow) typical of a vestibular schwannoma.

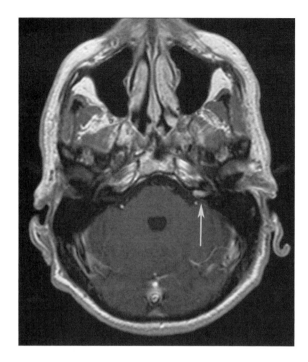

Figure P4.5

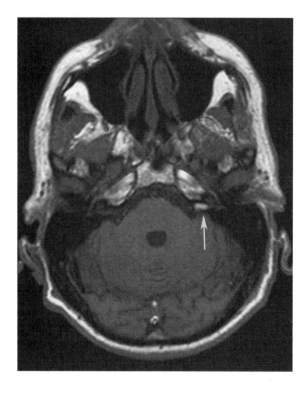

Figure P4.6

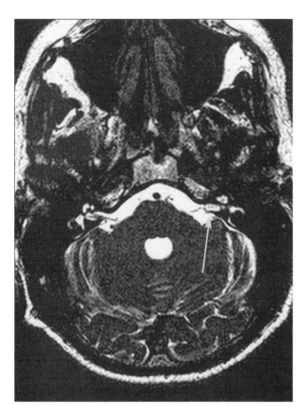

Figure P4.7

This axial T1WI with contrast (Figure P4.5) demonstrates high signal in the left IAC (arrow) from an IAC lipoma. While this may be mistaken for a vestibular schwannoma on a contrast exam, note that it looks nearly identical on the noncontrast T1WI (Figure P4.6, arrow). On the FIESTA scan (Figure P4.7) it disappears because it bright, just like CSF in the IAC which would not be expected with a solid schwannoma.

Pitfall 5

This 22-year-old college football player presented with severe headaches that persisted into the second week of his summer training. His doctor ordered a CT scan, which was followed by an MR scan with MRV (Figures P5.1–P5.3).

What is your leading diagnosis to explain the appearance of the transverse sinuses?

(1) a meningioma.

(2) a dural venous occlusion.

(3) an arachnoid granulation.

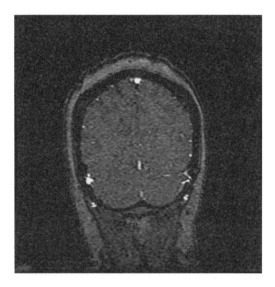

Figure P5.1

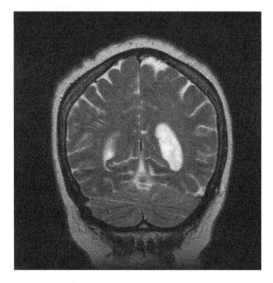

Figure P5.2

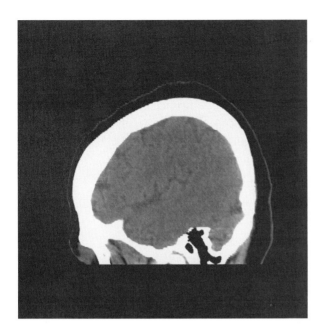

Figure P5.3

Correct answer: 3

PACCHIONIAN GRANULATIONS AND MRV

The findings are characteristic of a giant arachnoid granulation. These are normal variants that occur frequently in the transverse sinus, and for some reason they are more commonly seen on the left. One feature of the case that argues against an acute venous occlusion is that the density is too low on the CT scan and too bright on T2WI for an acute or even a subacute thrombus. Giant arachnoid granulations are quite common if you look for them (Figure P5.4) on vascular imaging studies and should not be mistaken for a dural sinus tumor or thrombus.

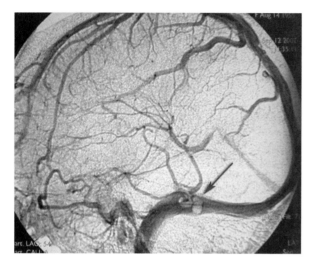

Figure P5.4 The venous phase of a cerebral angiogram from another patient shows the typical appearance of giant arachnoid granulations at the junction of the transverse and sigmoid sinuses (arrow). These never cause venous occlusion and usually appear as well defined intraluminal filling defects on vascular imaging.

Pitfall 6

This patient presented with persistent left ear pain. A temporal bone high resolution CT was obtained followed by an MR with contrast. With regard to the finding in the posterior left temporal bone as seen on the CT scan (Figure P6.1), FIESTA (Figure P6.2), and post contrast T1WI (Figure P6.3) your diagnosis is:

(1) chordoma.

(2) arachnoid granulation.

(3) endolymphatic sac tumor.

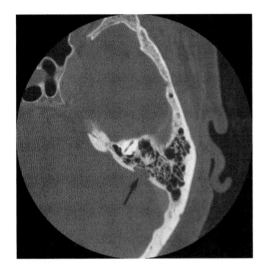

Figure P6.1

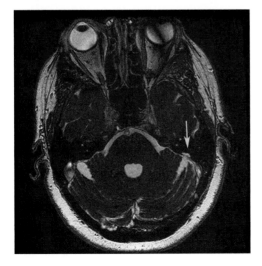

Figure P6.2

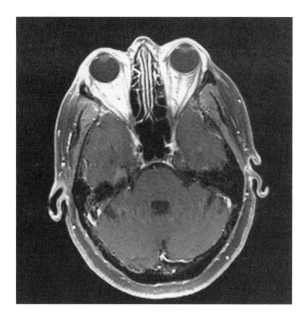

Figure P6.3

PETROUS BONE ARACHNOID GRANULATIONS

This is another arachnoid granulation, but it is an uncommon variation compared with the one in Pitfall 5. This particular CT finding of an erosion in the posterior petrous temporal bone also should suggest the diagnosis of an endolymphatic sac tumor, but the high signal on the axial FIESTA scan (Figure P6.2) and lack of enhancement (Figure P6.3) argue strongly against the diagnosis of a skull base tumor.

FIESTA is a steady state free precession (SSFP) gradient echo pulse sequence that uses the residual magnetization that persists between the repeated RF excitations to provide very high signal from fluid. This case illustrates the typical finding of this benign variation of anatomy which should not be mistaken for an endolymphatic sac tumor that may occur in this same region (Figures P6.4 and P6.5).

Correct answer: 3

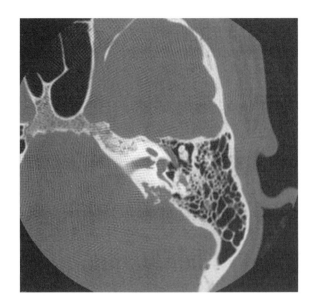

Figure P6.4

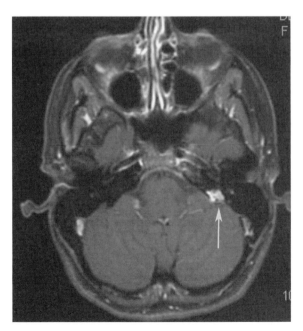

Figure P6.5

Here is a similar left petrous bone finding on CT (Figure P6.4) but the MR findings are different. The enhanced MR scan is abnormal in that same region which in this case was evidence of an endolymphatic tumor (Figure P6.5, arrow).

Pitfall 7

This 45-year-old male was scanned for persistant headache. The sagittal T1WI (Figure P7.1) demonstrates T1 shortening in the interhemispheric fissure (arrow) as well as a sellar and suprasellar mass. The most likely diagnosis to explain the bright midline signal in the falx is:

(1) metastatic disease.

(2) a ruptured dermoid.

(3) falx ossification.

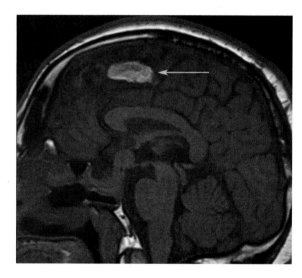

Figure P7.1

FALX OSSIFICATION

This is the typical appearance of fatty marrow with an ossified falx. You may be familiar with the high attenuation of the falx on CT due to calcification. It is common to see formation of bone, however, called ossification of the falx. As a result it can appear bright on T1WI because it contains fat in its marrow space. This fat is usually inapparent on CT because it is overwhelmed by the high attenuation of the calcification (Figure P7.2). It is only visible on MR because the calcified elements are now inapparent, so the short T1 of the marrow fat becomes more evident. In the setting of trauma, the differential diagnosis may include hemorrhage (Figures P7.3 and P7.4) and since CT is usually available this is usually not a difficult diagnosis. Fat suppressed images will confirm the nature of this signal (Figures P7.5 and P7.6). Remember that on diffusion-weighted imaging (DWI) acute blood and epidermoids may appear bright due to restricted diffusion, while fat will be suppressed since DWI scans are fat suppressed to eliminate chemical shift artifacts.

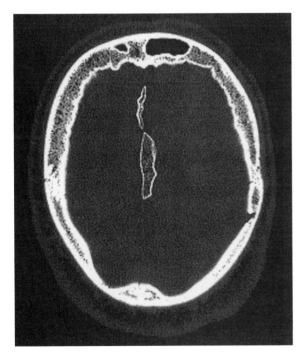

Figure P7.2 This axial CT scan reveals the cortex and marrow space in this ossified falx.

Correct answer: 3

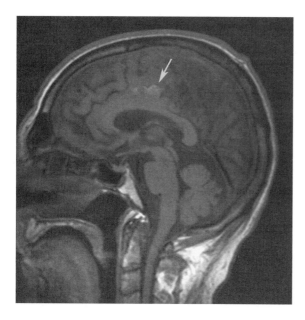

Figure P7.3

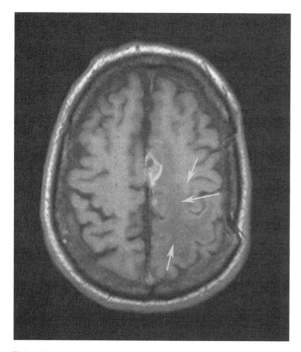

Figure P7.4

This patient shows evidence of T1 shortening in the midline but in this case from subarachnoid blood in the cingulate sulcus. Note that it is gyriform in contour on the sagittal view (Figure P7.3, arrow) and is associated with an adjacent brain abnormality on the axial scan (Figure P7.4, arrows).

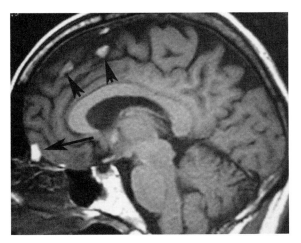

Figure P7.5

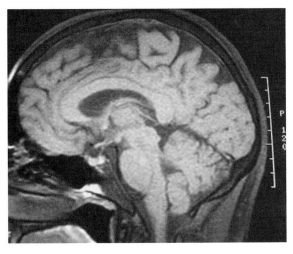

Figure P7.6

Figure P7.5 shows several areas midline high signal (arrowheads) which arises from fat in the falx, not hemorrhage, on this T1WI. If there is any question about that diagnosis, the observation that this signal vanishes on the chemical fat-suppressed image (Figure P7.6) confirms it. Also note that the high signal just above the ethmoid sinuses but below the frontal lobes (Figure 7.5, arrow) also disappears. This signal arises from the fat in the marrow space of the crista galli.

Pitfall 8

This 55-year-old male presents with a history of headaches that began 5 years ago. The glomus of the choroid plexus has this striking appearance on DWI (Figure P8.1) and FLAIR (Figure P8.2) imaging. What is your diagnosis?

(1) metastatic disease to the choroid plexus.

(2) bilateral choroid infection.

(3) benign neuroepithelial cysts.

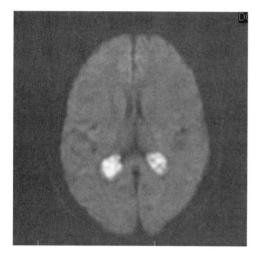

Figure P8.1

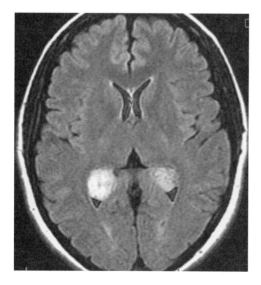

Figure P8.2

BRIGHT THINGS ON DIFFUSION

Choroid plexus cysts, also called neuroepithelial cysts, are not thought to be of any significance and are quite common with aging. It is important to not overreact to their high signal on DWI so that they are not mistaken for tumor or infection. One imaging feature that should allow you to make the correct diagnosis is that choroid plexus cysts do not show solid enhancement (Figures P8.3–P8.9), unlike tumors such as choroid plexus papilloma, metastatic disease, and intraventricular meningioma.

These cases are a reminder that not only infarcts can be bright on DWI. The source of the high signal on DWI with choroids cysts, much like that seen with epidermoids, is a composite of T2 shine through along with actual restricted diffusion.

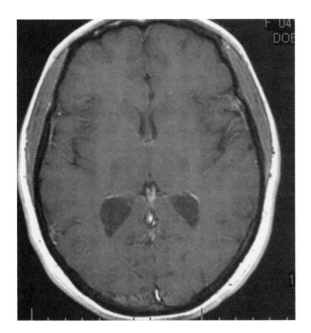

Figure P8.3 This postcontrast scan (Figure P8.3) from the same patient shown in Figure P8.1 shows no solid enhancement associated with the choroid masses.

Correct answer: 3

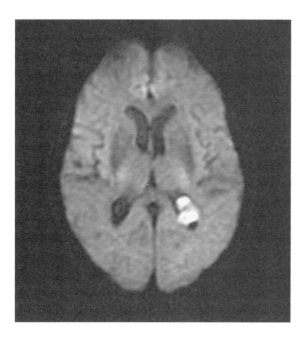

Figure P8.4

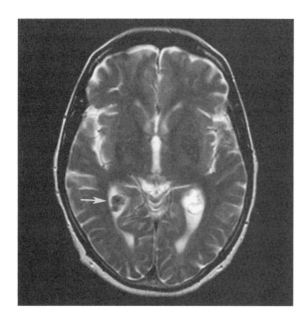

Figure P8.5

This diffusion scan (Figure P8.4) from another patient demonstrates a bright choroid but only on the left. The asymmetry in this case is due to a combination of low proton density and susceptibility effects in the right glomus due to calcification. Together they make it appear dark since diffusion is quite sensitive to susceptibility effects. The low proton density effect is more apparent on the T2WI (Figure P8.5, arrow).

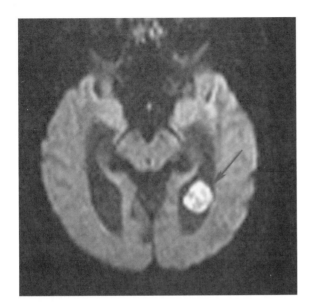

Figure P8.6

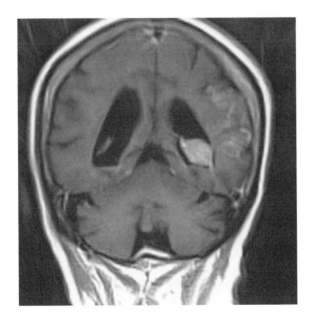

Figure P8.7

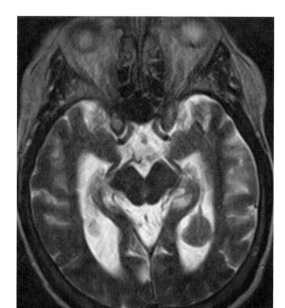

Figure P8.8

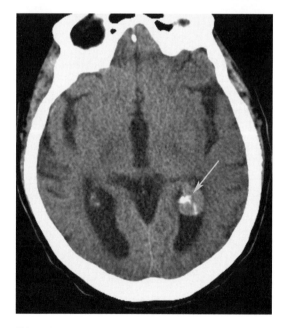

Figure P8.9

This patient presented with headaches as well. The diffusion scan (Figure P8.6) also shows a bright left glomus of the choroid plexus (arrow). The appearance on the contrast scan (Figure P8.7) and the T2WI scan (Figure P8.8), however, is not at all typical of benign neuroepithelial cysts since they do not enhance (see image P8.3). The findings considered together are most consistent with a tumor. While a xanthogranuloma of the choroid might be considered, the calcium on the CT scan (Figure 8.9, arrow), along with the homogeneous enhancement, best fits the diagnosis of intraventricular meningioma.

Pitfall 9

This 40-year-old male presents with symptoms that suggest MS. While you think that the spinal cord is normal, you notice a paraspinal mass with T2 prolongation (Figure P9.1, arrow) but no enhancement (Figure P9.2). Should you report this as:

(1) suspicious for a schwannoma?

(2) a lateral disc herniation?

(3) a duplication cyst?

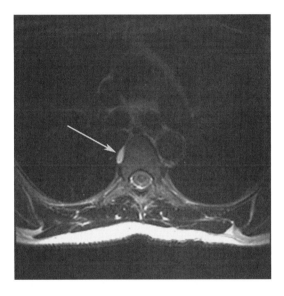

Figure P9.1

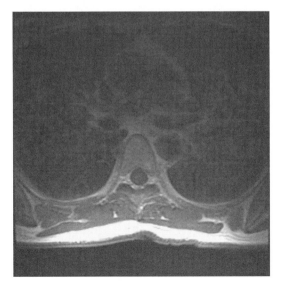

Figure P9.2

DUPLICATION CYSTS

While duplication cysts may be symptomatic, they are frequently discovered as incidental findings in adults. It is not uncommon to encounter them in the course of thoracic spine imaging. As a rule, no follow-up is necessary when they are asymptomatic and have characteristic MR findings of low signal on T1WI, uniformly high signal on T2WI, and no enhancement (Figures P9.3 and P9.4).

This pair of images using T1WI (Figure P9.5) and T2WI (Figure P9.6) illustrates a chemical shift artifact from another duplication cyst. Can we tell from these images the direction of phase encoding?

The dark line along the left anterior margin of this duplication cyst (Figure P9.6, arrows) indicates that the frequency shift is in the anterior-posterior direction, which, of course, means that the phase encoding direction must be from side to side.

Correct answer: 3

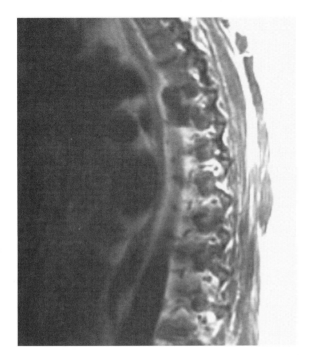

Figure P9.3

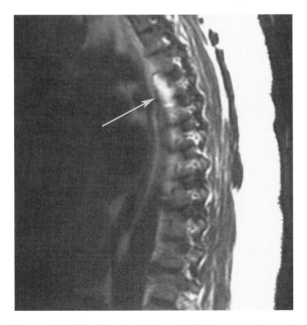

Figure P9.4

The sagittal T1WI with contrast (Figure P9.3) shows no evidence of enhancement of this duplication cyst, which is more evident on T2WI (Figure P9.4, arrow).

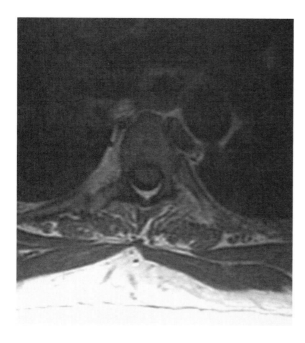

Figure P9.5

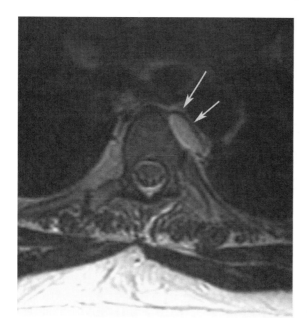

Figure P9.6

Pitfall 10

This 80-year-old patient presented with new headaches. Can you account for the midline dot of high signal on T1WI (Figure P10.1, arrow) that would also explain the streak artifacts on CT (Figure P10.2)?

(1) falx ossification.

(2) midline subarachnoid hemorrhage.

(3) Pantopaque.

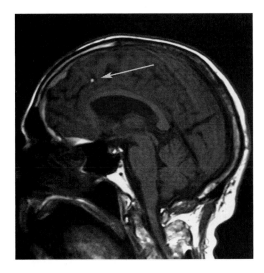

Figure P10.1

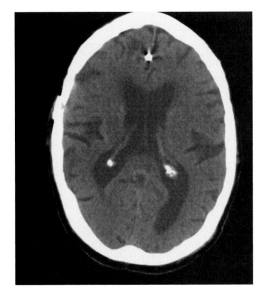

Figure P10.2

PANTOPAQUE ON MR

Ossification could explain the high signal on T1WI due to marrow and fat perhaps some high attenuation on CT due to cortical bone. However, streak artifacts indicate unusually high attenuation, higher than would be expected from calcium alone. The patient's age helps to make the diagnosis of retained Pantopaque in this case. The Pantopaque must have been left over from a myelogram performed some 30 years ago.

Pantopaque was a patented contast agent, an oil-ester, that was used for most myelograms over thirty years ago. When retained Pantopaque was imaged on MR it was found to demonstrate a short T1 and T2 relaxation time (Figures P10.3 and P10.4). When visualized in the spine, because of these imaging characteristics, it can easily be mistaken for hemorrhage.

Pantopaque replaced Lipiodol (iodinated poppyseed oil) as a CNS contrast agent and was in common use for myelography from 1944 to the late 1970's. It was quickly replaced, however, when a suitable water soluble contrast agent (Metrizimide) was approved for this application in 1973.

This rapid transition to water soluble contrast agents was due in part to the fact that the use of Pantopaque for myelography required a specific and demanding technique. After it was instilled into the subarachnoid space and the appropriate films obtained, it had to be removed by careful aspiration through a large-gauge spinal needle. This was because of legitimate concerns about residual contrast inciting arachnoiditis. While some argued at the time that Pantopaque would be resorbed at a predictable rate, the fact that it may still be evident on imaging some 30 years later suggests that this was not always the case (Figures P10.5 and P10.6).

Correct answer: 3

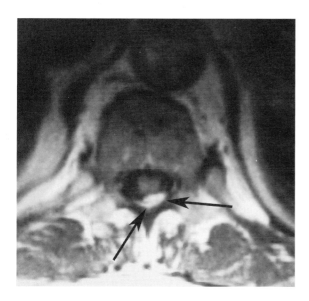

Figure P10.3

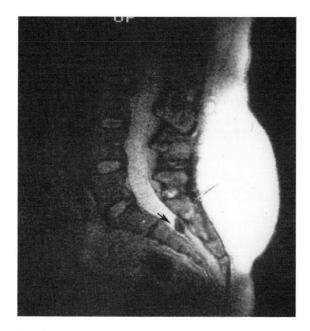

Figure P10.4

These images demonstrate the typical appearance of Pantopaque on MR. Note the high signal on T1WI (arrow, Figure P10.3) and the fluid-fluid level on T2WI, where the low-signal Pantopaque layers (short T2 relaxation time) with the bright CSF (long T2 relaxation time) in the dependent lumbar canal (arrow, Figure P10.4).

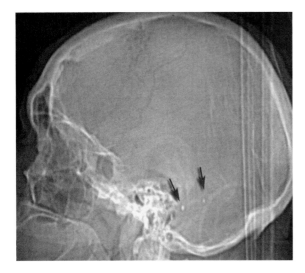

Figure P10.5

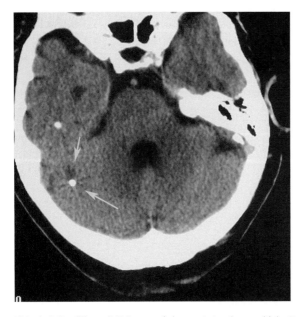

Figure P10.6

This skull film (Figure P10.5, arrows) demonstrates the very high attenuation of Pantopaque. The stellate dark lines around it on the CT scan (Figure P10.6, arrows) are due to photon starvation since pantopaque in a sense creates x-ray shadows because its attenuation factor is so high. This appearance helps to establish the diagnosis since calcium would not be expected to create these streak artifacts.

Pitfall 11

This 45-year-old man presented to the hospital with confusion and symptoms of severe sepsis. Shortly after admission, his respiratory symptoms worsened and he required intubation. On his third hospital day he was brought to the MR suite for a brain scan. On the FLAIR scan his CSF appeared diffusely abnormal with increased signal in the subarachnoid space (Figures P11.1 and P11.2). A spinal tap was performed but was normal. How can you explain the FLAIR findings?

(1) flow artifacts.

(2) oxygen effects.

(3) improper selection of scan TR or TI times.

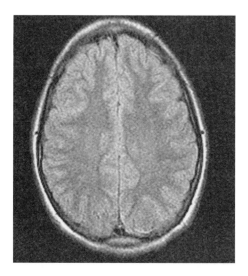

Figure P11.1

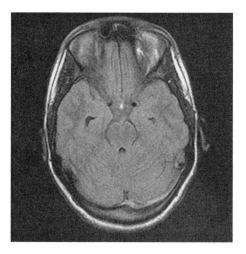

Figure P11.2

OXYGEN EFFECTS ON FLAIR

The CSF appears to be diffusely abnormal, with no visible sulci, on Figures P11.1 and P11.2. The signal from the CSF in the temporal horn, however, is suppressed, suggesting that the imaging parameters were entered correctly. This appearance. Which suggests diffuse disease of the subarachnoid space, may be seen in patients receiving supplemental inhaled oxygen. This pitfall was noted early on when FLAIR was incorporated into routine imaging, and it was initially attributed to the anesthetic agents frequently used to image sick patients and children. Eventually, it became apparent that oxygen alone could explain this appearance.

Oxygen is a paramagnetic agent, and once the concentration of dissolved oxygen is high enough in the blood serum, it will increase in the CSF as well. Low-flow inhaled oxygen using nasal prongs is usually not sufficient to explain this appearance; it is most often seen in patients who are intubated.

There are other reasons why the CSF can appear diffusely abnormal when it is in fact normal. If a patient, with or without renal insufficiency, has an MR scan of the brain within 24 to 48 hours after receiving an IV gadolinium contrast agent, the gadolinium can appear in the CSF. As a result of this T1 shortening, an abnormal appearance of the CSF will be evident on FLAIR. This effect may be particularly prominent in patients in whom the meninges are diseased, since the IV contrast weeps into the subarachnoid space from the abnormal meninges. On those occasions, the gadolinium effect may be both intense and focal (Figure P11.3).

You may be wondering why these gadolinium and oxygen T1 effects are not evident on T1WI images. This is because FLAIR is much more sensitive than T1WI to alterations of T1 relaxation of CSF.

Correct answer: 3

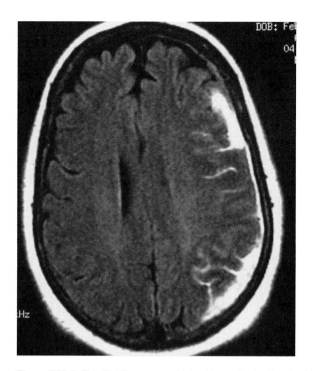

Figure P11.3 This FLAIR scan was obtained in a patient with a dural-based metastatic lesion. After he received gadolinium, the tumor enhanced but abnormal signal was also evident in the nearby subarachnoid space on this postcontrast scan. This appearance is due to T1 shortening of CSF in the subarachnoid space from contrast weeping into the subarachnoid space from the abnormal dural surface.

Pitfall 12

This 40-year-old male presented with increasing lethargy after several days of fever. Here is the axial FLAIR image (Figure P12.1) and the corresponding T2WI (Figure P12.2). Do you think his FLAIR scan is abnormal? If so, where?

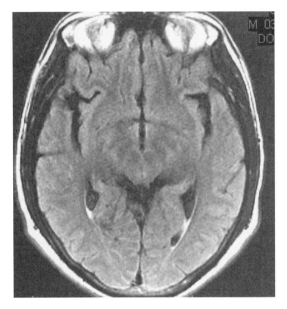

Figures P12.1

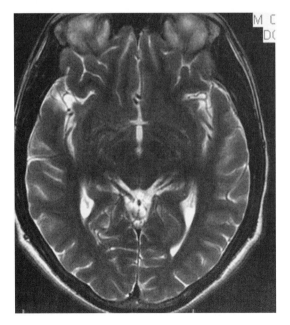

Figure P12.2

This patient proved to have meningitis. While his FLAIR image (Figure P12.1) does not show diffusely bright cortical sulci, the absence of visible sulci in the medial occipital lobes, along with the patient's history, is sufficient to suggest that diagnosis.

Because of the suppression of signal from normal CSF, the ventricles and the entire subarachnoid space should appear dark. While focal abnormalities can be quite evident (see Pitfall 11), usually the most difficult cases to identify as abnormal have diffuse, symmetric findings. In this case, the subarachnoid space in the cortical sulci is isointense with adjacent normal brain in the medial occipital lobes, while the CSF appears dark in other spaces such as the sylvian fissures. At times, however, this appearance can be normal if the gyri are swollen and the cortical sulci are effaced. One method to help establish how the cortical sulci should appear on the FLAIR scan is to look at the FLAIR image next to the corresponding T2WI (Figure P12.3). The abnormalities are particularly evident after the image contrast is reversed on the T2WI (usually a one click option on a computer workstation). Consider performing this comparison to detect any sulci on FLAIR that do not match with corresponding dark sulci on the reversed T2WI (Figures P12.4–P12.6).

Full suppression of the CSF depends somewhat on scanner settings, so it is possible to make normal CSF look isointense with brain on the basis of image technique alone. The tipoff that the absent sulci are due to the imaging parameters is that the CSF in the ventricles may appear isointense with brain as well, a pattern that is almost never seen with subarachnoid hemorrhage, meningitis, or inhaled oxygen (Figures P12.7 and P12.8).

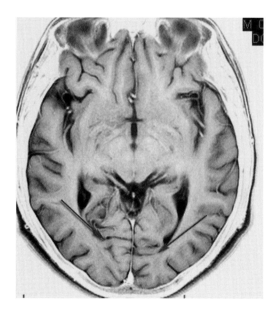

Figure P12.3 The axial FLAIR scan (Figure P12.1) from this case has missing sulci in the medial occipital lobes that becomes evident when it is compared with the corresponding slice on a reversed T2WI (Figure P12.3, arrows).

Correct answer: Abnormal subarachnoid spaces, medial occipital lobes.

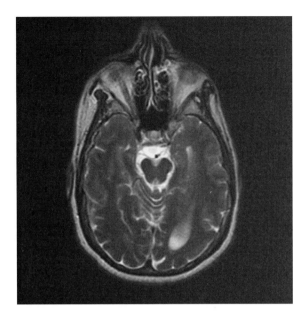

Figure P12.4

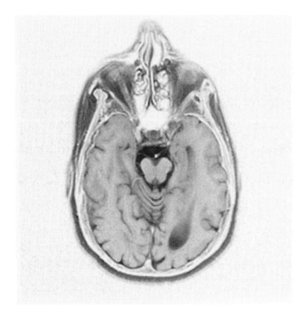

Figure P12.5

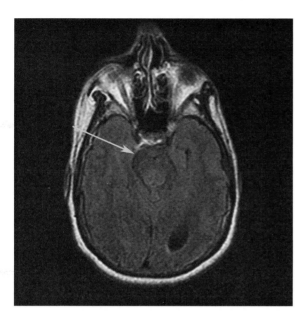

Figure P12.6

Here is another example of a T2WI (Figure P12.4), the reversed T2WI (Figure P12.5), and the corresponding FLAIR scan (Figure P12.6). This case has more obvious abnormalities of the subarachnoid space with blurring of the basilar cisterns (Figure P12.6, arrow) and cortical sulci diffusely on the FLAIR image.

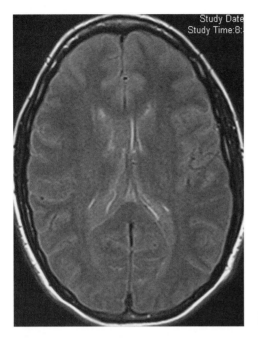

Figure P12.7

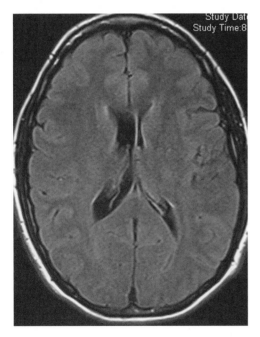

Figure P12.8

These images from two FLAIR scans of the same patient were obtained within minutes of each other. In Figure P12.7 (using TR 6000) all the CSF, both intraventricular and over the convexities, is isointense with the brain, while Figure P12.8 (TR 10,000) shows the normal low signal of CSF in those same spaces. The signal intensity of CSF is influenced by flow, TR, TI, and overall magnet homogeneity, so the extent of CSF signal suppression may vary among scanners and different techniques.

Pitfall 13

This MRV was obtained urgently in a newborn with seizures. Based on this image (Figure P13.1), you think that this patient has:

(1) normal venous drainage of the brain.

(2) thrombosis of the deep venous system but a normal superior sagittal sinus.

(3) thrombosis of both the deep and superficial venous systems.

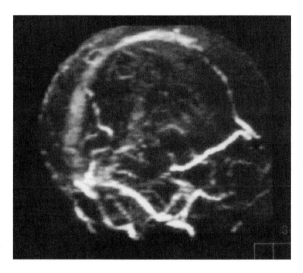

Figure P13.1

SHINE THROUGH ON TOF MRA

Shine through of subacute thrombus is an important pitfall and is common to all TOF MRA imaging. The bright intravascular signal on TOF MRA is due to entry slice enhancement, but anything with a short T1 relaxation time, such as fat or thrombus, will also appear bright on these gradient images and this effect is called "shine through". This is because 2D TOF MRA uses a rapidly repeating RF pulse to suppress background signal in order to increase the contrast between static tissue and the high signal arising from moving blood. However, if the T1 relaxation time of the static tissue is sufficiently short, it will also appear bright on the image and resemble flow-related enhancement on the MIP (Figure P13.2).

Shine through may also be evident on 3D TOF images, where it is common to see some orbital fat or even the posterior pituitary if you look carefully (Figure P13.3). Shine through in MRA can be problematic, however, if the patient has a lipoma near a vessel that is mistaken for vascular pathology on the MIP reconstructions. For this reason, you should not rely on TOF MRA for diagnosis without obtaining at least one T1WI (Figures P13.4–P13.6).

This pitfall can be avoided by using phase contrast MRV as a replacement for or in addition to a 2D TOF MRV. The value of this sequence, even though it may be more challenging to interpret at times, is that all of the high signal arises entirely from the movement of hydrogen protons so shine through of subacute thrombus is never a question (Figures P13.7 and P13.8).

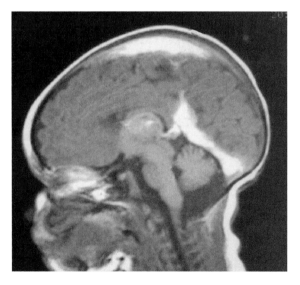

Figure P13.2 This sagittal T1WI demonstrates abnormal high signal in the deep and superficial cerebral veins and sinuses consistent with subacute thrombosis. As a result of this T1 shortening, the venous system may appear to have flow on the 2D TOF MRV, an artifact called shine through.

Correct answer: 3

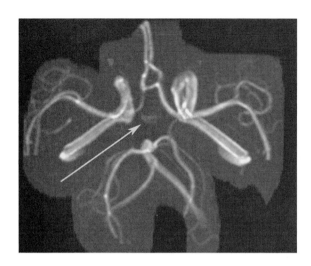

Figure P13.3 The collapsed view from a 3D TOF MRA of a patient with a normal intracranial circulation shows a small area of high signal at the midline (arrow) representing the posterior pituitary, which appears (*shines through)* because of its short T1 relaxation time.

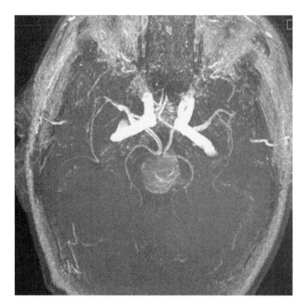

Figure P13.4

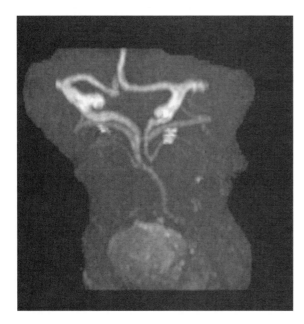

Figure P13.5

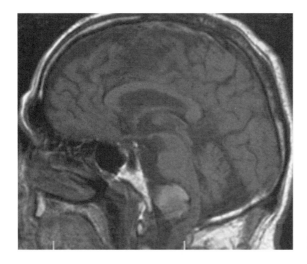

Figure P13.6

The axial (Figure P13.4) and the coronal MIP of the posterior circulation (Figure P13.5) demonstrate what appears to be flow-related enhancement of a large aneurysm at the skull base. The sagittal T1WI (Figure P13.6) demonstrates that this skull base mass is bright not from flow but rather T1 shortening from a blood clot in this large thrombosed aneurysm. Note that the orbital fat is also visible on this 3D TOF exam (Figure P13.4), another example of shine through and a reminder that high signal on TOF imaging may not indicate flow.

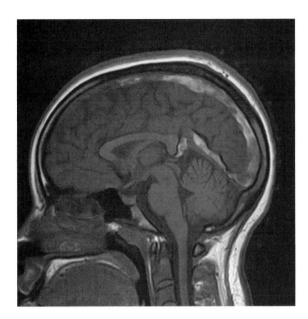

Figure P13.7

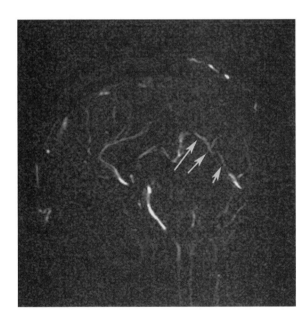

Figure P13.8

This sagittal T1WI (Figure P13.7) reveals dural sinus thrombosis with high signal in the SSS and clot in the deep system as well. The phase contrast MRV (Figure P13.8) shows a small channel in the straight sinus (arrows) from recanalization, but there is no flow in the superior sagittal sinus. Phase contrast MRA images may be harder to read than 2D TOF images, however, because it is usually quite difficult to recognize that something is missing since only patent vessels are visible.

Pitfall 14

This 35-year-old male presented with a history of headaches. His MR scans demonstrate asymmetric, abnormal signal in the right petrous apex. The axial T1WI (Figure P14.1, arrow), FLAIR (Figure P14.2, arrow), diffusion (Figure P14.3), and T2WI (Figure P14.4) are available for your review. You believe that this finding represents:

   (1) a congenital cholesteotoma.

   (2) a giant cholesterol cyst.

   (3) nothing to worry about.

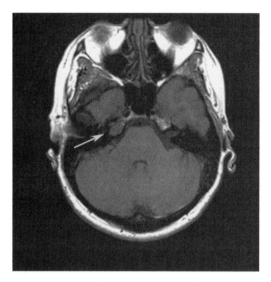

Figure P14.1

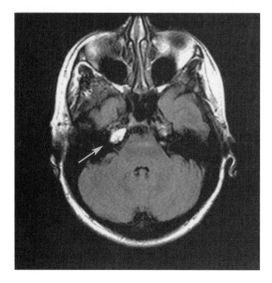

Figure P14.2

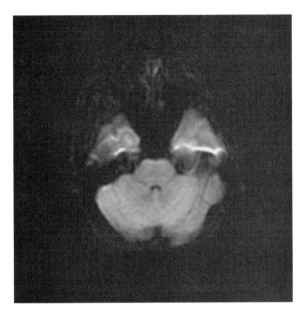

Figure P14.3

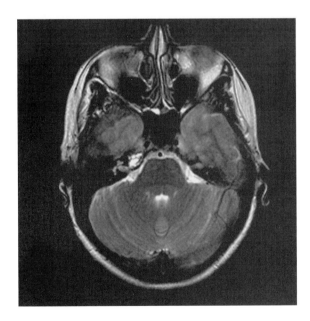

Figure P14.4

LEAVE ME ALONE PETROUS APEX LESIONS

The signal in the petrous apex reflects fluid within medial mastoid air cells and has no clinical significance. It becomes significant in a negative way, however, when someone suggests that it could represent a tumor or an infection. In cases where concerns persist, a CT scan should prove valuable by showing normal, albeit opacified, medial air cells (Figures P14.5 and P14.6) but without bony destruction (Figures P14.7 and P14.8). While this is also the typical location for a giant cholesterol cyst, that lesion should be bright on T1WI (Figures P14.9–P14.11).

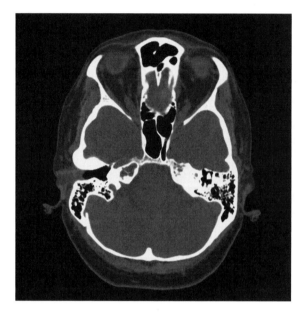

Figure P14.5

Correct answer: 3

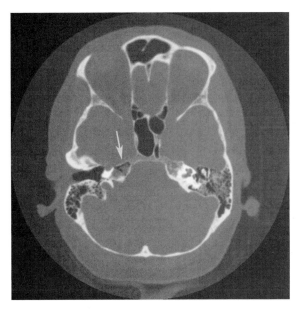

Figure P14.6

This patient had a CT scan (Figure P14.5) near the time of the MR and a repeat CT scan 1 month later. These scans show no bony destruction or expansion in the right petrous bone but the medial air cells have intermediate attenuation indicating fluid. Note that there is partial clearing of the fluid on the later exam (Figure P14.6, arrow).

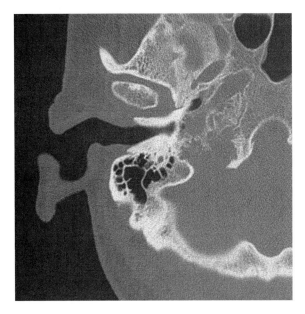

Figure P14.7

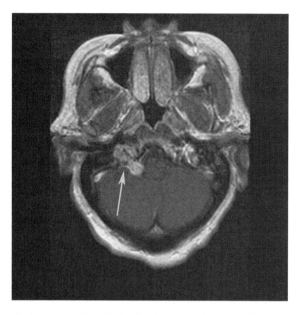

Figure P14.8

The CT scan of this patient with a glomus jugulare tumor shows bony destructive changes involving the right jugular bulb (Figure P14.7) corresponding to the enhancing mass on MR (Figure P14.8, arrow).

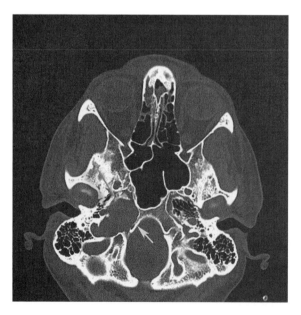

Figure P14.9

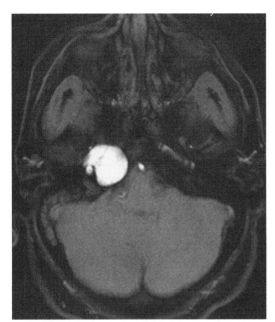

Figure P14.10

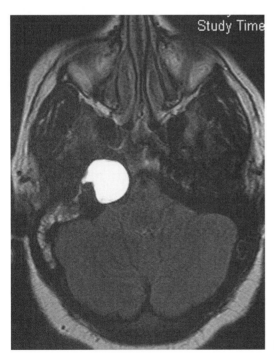

Study Time

Figure P14.11

This diagnosis of a giant cholesterol cyst can be established in this case on the basis of the smooth bone remodeling on CT (Figure P14.9, arrow), T1 shortening (seen here on a fat-suppressed scan, Figure P14.10), and abnormal high signal on the FLAIR scan (Figure P14.11).

Pitfall 15

This 25-year-old female presents with new headaches. She had a previous MR exam at another center, where a pineal mass was identified and reported as a pineal cyst. You request that her new MR scan include three planes (axial, coronal, sagittal) T1WI postcontrast. Figure P15.1 is her sagittal postcontrast T1WI. After seeing this abnormal signal in the pineal region (arrow), should you ask:

(1) for the phone so that you can call neurosurgery?

(2) when this sagittal T1WI scan was obtained?

(3) for imaging of the entire spine to look for a drop metastasis?

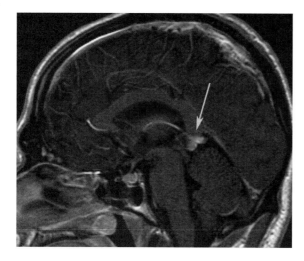

Figure P15.1

PINEAL CYST ENHANCEMENT

Pineal cysts are quite common and occur more frequently in women than in men. They prove to be troublesome on imaging because they do not behave like arachnoid cysts i.e. arachnoid cysts usually suppress on FLAIR and do not enhance. Pineal cysts are not necessarily filled with clear CSF because they do not communicate freely with the subarachnoid space or the ventricle in most cases. This would explain why the fluid within pineal cysts does not usually suppress on FLAIR imaging (Figure P15.2). Contrast-enhanced imaging is helpful when you are trying to differentiate a pineal cyst from a pineocytoma since the latter should have a solidly enhancing nodule. But if you decide to administer contrast, it is important to keep in mind that the normal pineal gland does not have a blood-brain barrier. That is why you should expect to see some rim enhancement in the wall of any benign pineal cyst (Figure P15.3).

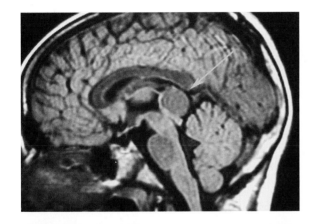

Figure P15.2

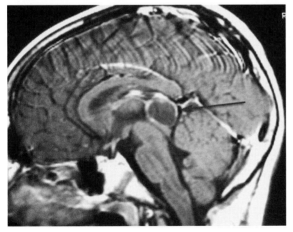

Figure P15.3

This sagittal T1WI (Figure P15.2) of a patient with a large, benign pineal cyst (arrow) shows that the cyst contents differ in signal from the CSF on this sagittal FLAIR scan. That is because the fluid in a pineal cyst may contain protein or even blood. The enhanced T1WI (Figure P15.3) from the same patient demonstrates the expected rim of enhancement since the pineal gland, which makes up the wall of the cyst, has no blood-brain barrier (arrow).

Correct answer: 2

While this rim enhancement is typical, if there is a delay after the contrast is given or if multiple postcontrast scans are acquired, enough time may elapse for the contrast to leak from the normal enhancing pineal tissue into the cyst fluid. This can occasionally make a benign rim-enhancing pineal cyst resemble a solidly enhancing mass. In this particular case, the sagittal scan was obtained last. If you look carefully, you can actually see the contrast-fluid level from contrast collecting in the dependent pineal cyst fluid.

If you add a sagittal FIESTA or other high-resolution scan to your imaging protocol for pineal cysts, be careful that you do not mistake structure in the cyst as evidence of an underlying tumor. While many benign pineal cysts have a smooth rim, you should not be surprised to find that many others have some degree of fine internal structure (Figure P15.4, arrow).

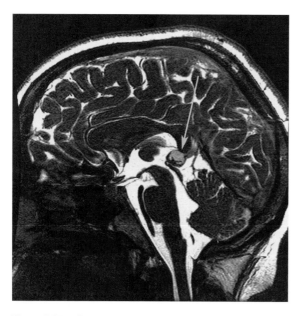

Figure P15.4 Sagittal FIESTA image of a benign pineal cyst. The fine internal structure and irregular wall should not be mistaken for evidence of an underlying tumor. It is just a reflection of the resolution of this scan technique that can provide submillimeter slice thickness with high contrast at a tissue-fluid interface.

Pitfall 16

This patient has a history of headaches and right-sided third nerve palsy. Abnormal sections from her CT scan (Figure P16.1) and 2D TOF MRA scan (Figure P16.2) are available. On the basis of these images, do you think that this patient has:

(1) a large cavernous aneurysm?

(2) a meningioma?

(3) a fifth nerve schwannoma?

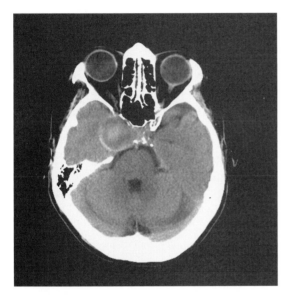

Figure P16.1

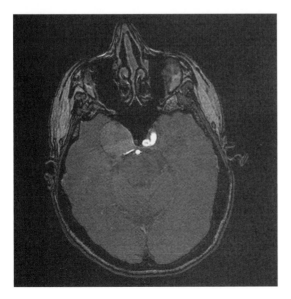

Figure P16.2

SLOW VASCULAR FLOW ON 3D TOF MRA

This case illustrates a potential pitfall of 3D TOF MRA imaging, i.e., the atypical appearance of aneurysms due to slow flow. That is because vascular imaging on 3D TOF MRA depends on rapid blood flow. While in this case the TOF scan (Figure P16.2) shows the expected high signal of the normal left carotid flow, the large aneurysm sac appears nearly isointense with nearby static brain. Computed tomographic angiography (CTA) has considerable value in such cases because it is not dependent on flow velocity to create contrast (Figures P16.3 and P16.4). I often hear radiologists add to their MRA reports that "small aneurysms may be missed on MRA" but they should also say that "large, slow flow aneurysms may be missed as well" to be perfectly accurate.

Correct answer: 1

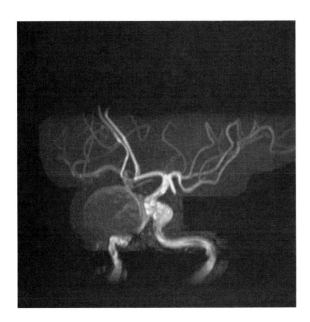

Figure P16.3

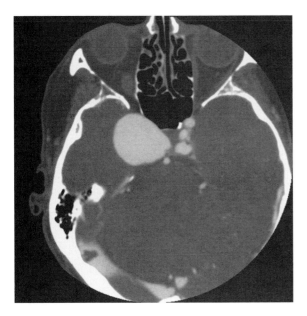

Figure P16.4

This MIP reconstruction (Figure P16.3) from the 2DTOF scan reveals very little flow-related enhancement within this large right cavernous aneurysm. The CTA, however (Figure P16.4), nicely demonstrates the lumen of this aneurysm because vascular contrast enhancement on CTA is based only on the timing of contrast arrival and the inherent high attenuation of the contrast, not on flow velocity.

Pitfall 17

This 45-year-old male with a history of spine surgery presents with new bilateral arm symptoms. His axial sagittal T1WI (Figure P17.1) and axial gradient echo scan (Figure P17.2) demonstrate:

(1) severe spinal stenosis.

(2) a large disc-osteophyte complex.

(3) a normal canal.

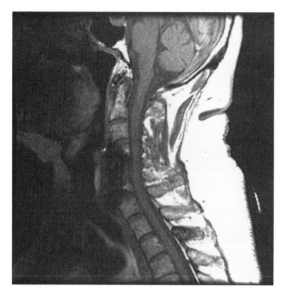

Figure P17.1

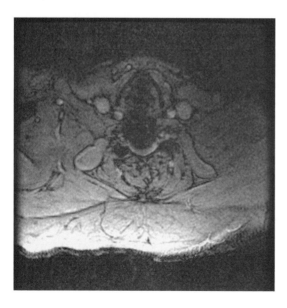

Figure P17.2

The appearance of the cervical canal on the axial FSE T2WI (Figure P17.3) corresponds more closely to its appearance on the sagittal T1WI (Figure P17.1), and both show no evidence of cord compression. The discrepancy between the FSE T2WI and the axial gradient echo scan (Figure P17.2) reflects their relative sensitivity to metal artifact. Fast spin echo T2WI is quite insensitive to susceptibility effects largely because it uses a 180 degree pulse to create an echo. The gradient echo scan (Figure P17.2) suggests a severe canal stenosis, but this appearance in fact reflects the magnetic field distortion due to artifacts from the hardware placed at surgery that is exaggerated by the use of a gradient echo technique for signal collection.

Metal artifacts after surgery in the cervical spine are particularly evident when metal plates or screws are used for stabilization. In some cases, however, a significant metal artifact may be apparent on MR after cervical diskectomy, while the plain films appear to be normal. This is attributed to flakes of metal that remain in the bone after a drill is used on the bony cortex. While small enough to be invisible on routine radiographs, this residual metal creates sufficient susceptibility effect to be evident on MR. That is the reason that FSE T2WI should be used in patients after spine surgery if accurate depiction of the canal anatomy is necessary. This is important to keep in mind anytime artifacts from metal are anticipated on MR (Figures P17.4 and P17.5).

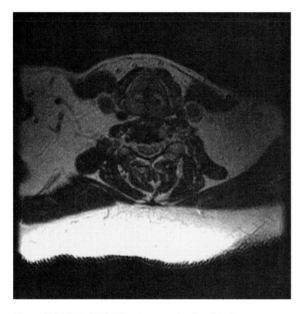

Figure P17.3 Axial T2WI at the same level as P17.2.

Correct answer: 3

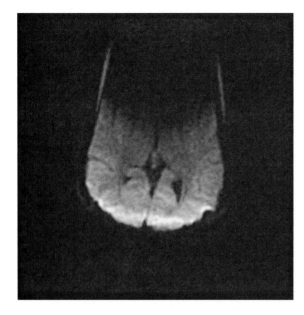

Figure P17.4

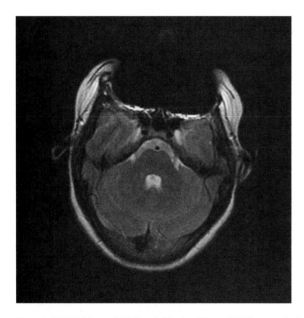

Figure P17.5

The axial T2WI (Figure P17.4) and diffusion (Figure P17.5) scans both demonstrate distortion due to metal braces in the patient's mouth. The artifact is more conspicuous on the diffusion exam (Figure P17.5) than T2WI because the diffusion study uses an echo planar technique that is more sensitive to magnetic susceptibility effects.

Pitfall 18

This patient with a history of lung cancer presented for a staging MR scan with the indication "rule out metastatic disease." The patient was reluctant to receive contrast but proceeded with the rest of the MR scan. In your view, this normal appearing FLAIR scan (Figure P18.1):

(1) makes it so unlikely that she has brain metastatic disease that contrast is not necessary.

(2) while it is normal it doesn't exclude metastatic disease to the brain.

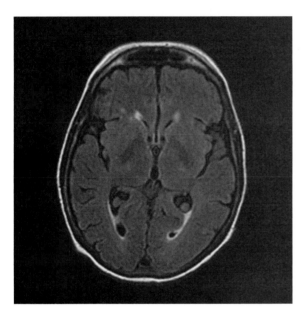

Figure P18.1

ROLE OF CONTRAST WITH BRAIN METASTATIC DISEASE

Even with the two images (Figures P18.1 and P18.2) side by side, you would be hard pressed to find any of these enhancing lesions on the FLAIR scan, and there is no chance that you could identify any of them as metastatic lesions on the FLAIR scan without the contrast images. While vasogenic edema is considered a typical feature of metastatic disease, you cannot rely on seeing edema with all metastatic lesions to the brain (Figures P18.3–P18.8).

When there is a question of metastatic disease in any patient with a history of cancer, contrast is necessary to fully evaluate the brain (Figure P18.5–P18.8). The answer to the question "How many metastatic lesions are in the brain?" is more complex because their conspicuity is influenced by scan technique, contrast dosage, and time elapsed from administration of contrast to performance of the scan. While more lesions become more evident by optimizing the technique (often at the expense of specificity), it is not always clear how to use this information in a treatment algorithm that may have been based on routine MR imaging or even enhanced CT.

One approach to increasing the sensitivity to brain metastatic lesions is to utilize an MR technique with higher sensitivity for contrast enhancement, such as magnetization transfer, and wait 20 minutes after administration of contrast (Figures P18.9–P18.11) to allow more contrast to leak into the brain since there should be no blood brain barrier in metastatic lesions.

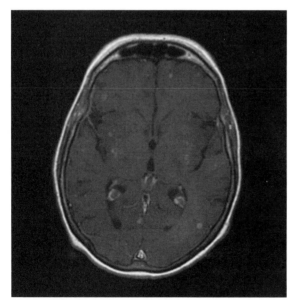

Figure P18.2 Postcontrast T1WI at the same level as Figure P18.1.

Correct answer: 2

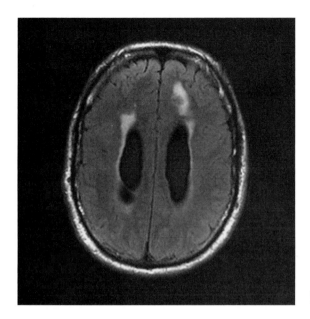

Figure P18.3

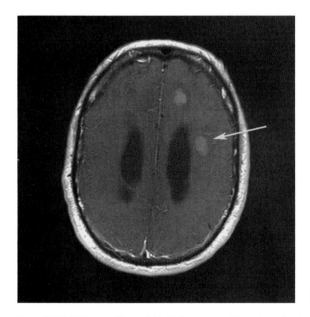

Figure P18.4

The axial FLAIR image (Figure P18.3) shows some T2 prolongation in the left frontal lobe that corresponds to one brain metastasis, but it appears completely normal where the second metastasis is demonstrated on the postcontrast scan at the same level (Figure P18.4, arrow).

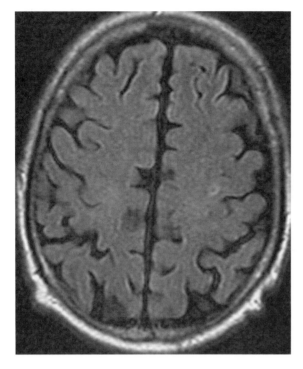

Figure P18.5

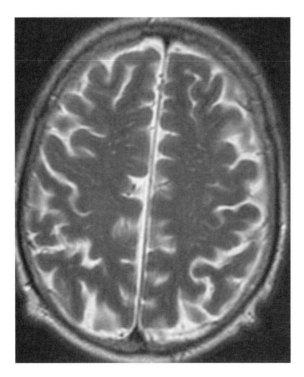

Figure P18.6

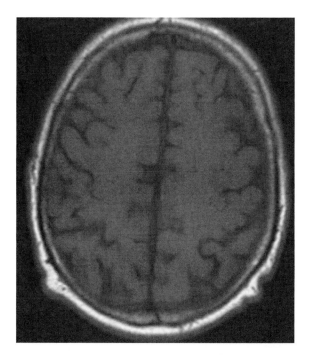

Figure P18.7

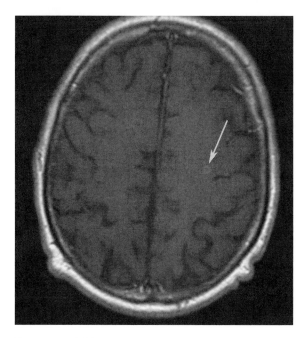

Figure P18.8

The axial FLAIR (Figure P18.5), T2WI (Figure P18.6), and T1WI (Figure P18.7) illustrate the limitations of any number of noncontrast MR scans for identification of this single enhancing metastatic lesion seen here on postcontrast T1WI (Figure P18.8, arrow).

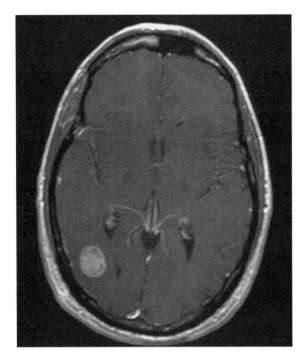

Figure P18.9

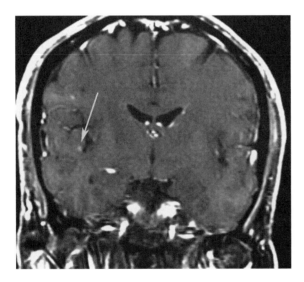

Figure P18.10

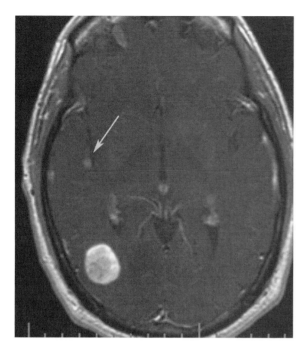

Figure P18.11

The axial (Figure P18.9) and coronal (Figure P18.10) post contrast T1WIs demonstrate at least one metastasis, but the second lesion (Figure P18.10, arrow), while visible on all the scans, is much more conspicuous on this delayed, post contrast axial T1 MT scan (Figure P18.11, arrow), that was obtained after a 10-minute delay from the time of contrast administration.

Pitfall 19

This patient presents with chronic headaches. The most likely diagnosis to explain the findings in the midbrain (Figures P19.1–P19.3) (arrow) is:

(1) primary brain tumor.

(2) cavernous malformation.

(3) giant perivascular space.

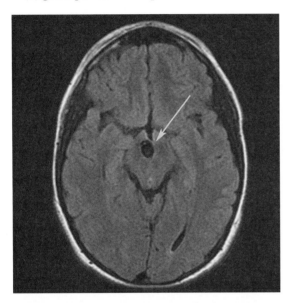

Figure P19.1

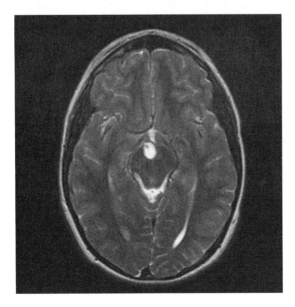

Figure P19.2

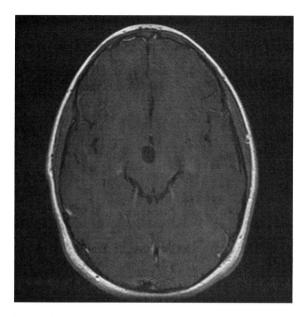

Figure P19.3

Axial FLAIR (Figure P19.1), T2WI (Figure P19.2), and T1WI with contrast (Figure P19.3) are at the same level in the brain of this patient with headaches.

GIANT PERIVASCULAR SPACES

The Virchow-Robin spaces, or perivascular spaces, surround the cerebral vasculature and extend to the subarachnoid space. While generally quite small, they may become particularly evident when they enlarge with age or after head trauma. Nevertheless, they have little clinical significance because it is not uncommon to find large perivascular spaces at any age. They may be large or unusually evident in one region of the brain without any clear cause. These are often found in the region of the midbrain, basal ganglia (Figure P19.4), and centrum semiovale (Figures P19.5 and P19.6). On occasion they can become quite large, but as long as they behave like CSF on FLAIR imaging, do not enhance, and are evident in these typical locations, you should feel comfortable calling them benign perivascular spaces.

Theses lesions provide another example of how the sensitivity of FLAIR imaging in detecting subtle changes in the composition of CSF can be helpful. The reason for this sensitivity is that the addition of even a small amount of blood or protein to the CSF will alter its relaxation time sufficiently that the net magnetization of the involved CSF will not arrive squarely on the zero axis at the moment when the 90 degree pulse arrives. It is very unusual for a tumor cyst in a high grade glial tumor or metastatic lesion to completely suppress on FLAIR for this reason.

Correct answer: 3

On rare occasions, clusters of giant perivascular spaces may appear in one location accompanied by mild mass effect and for this reason it resembles a cystic brain tumor. More troublesome, in some of these cases you may even find slight T2 prolongation surrounding the cysts on FLAIR (Figures P19.7–P19.9). This appearance on MR is called *tumefactive perivascular spaces*. In this circumstance it is important to consider this diagnosis although follow up imaging may be prudent depending on your confidence level.

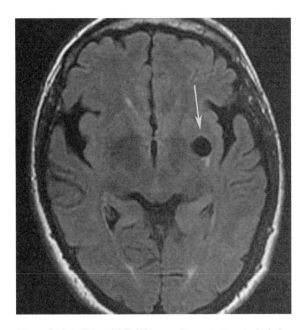

Figure P19.4 This axial FLAIR scans demonstrates a typical giant perivascular space in the region of the inferior putamen (arrow).

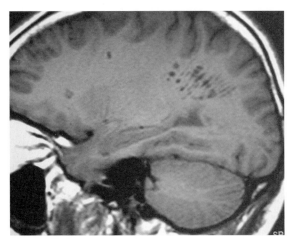

Figure P19.5

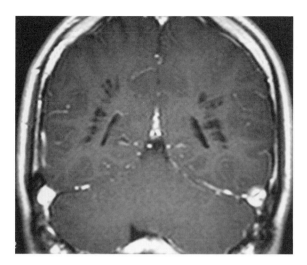

Figure P19.6

These images demonstrate multiple but typical enlarged perivascular spaces in the white matter on T1WI (Figure P19.5) and enhanced T1WI (Figure P19.6).

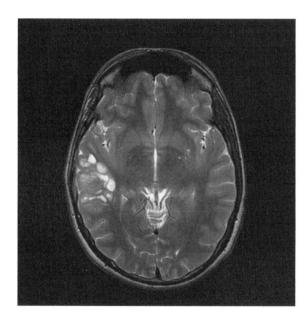

Figure P19.7

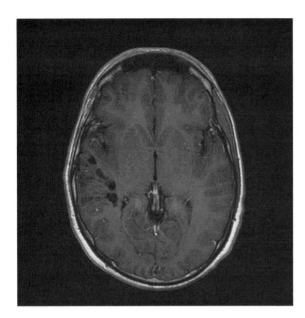

Figure P19.8

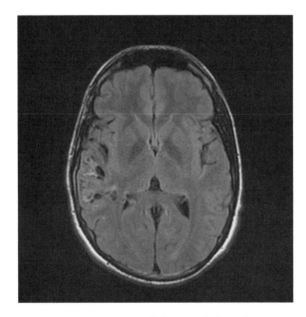

Figure P19.9

This case illustrates findings typical for tumefactive perivascular spaces based on the sharply defined cysts on T2WI (Figure P19.7),no enhancement after IV constrast (Figure P19.8), and suppression of cyst fluid (Figure P19.9) although there is some linear T2 prolongation that is evident on FLAIR imaging.

Pitfall 20

These axial T2WI (Figure P20.1), T1WI (Figure P20.2), and FLAIR (Figure P20.3) are most compatible with the diagnosis of:

   (1) a primary brain tumor.

   (2) an aneurysm.

   (3) a cavernoma.

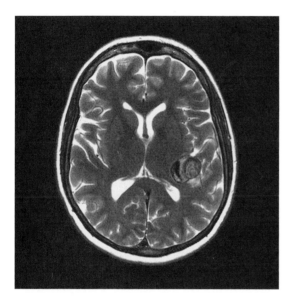

Figure P20.1

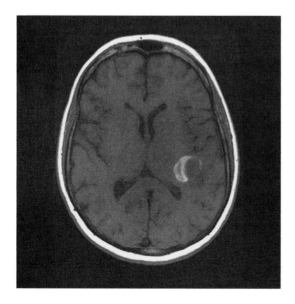

Figure P20.2

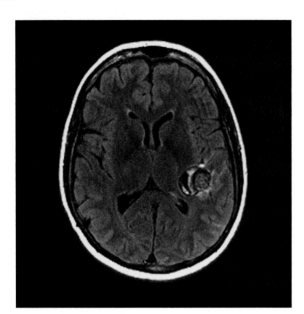

Figure P20.3

CEREBRAL ANEURYSM RESEMBLING A CAVERNOMA

While a circumferential dark border on T2WI is typical of cavernous malformations, it is not specific for that diagnosis since aneurysms may also have this appearance. It is important to recognize that this lesion, which at first glance appears to be an intra-parenchymal lesion, is located at the posterior sylvian fissure and is in fact extra-axial. A CTA scan was obtained for that reason; it established the diagnosis of a partially thrombosed, fusiform aneurysm of the left middle cerebral artery (Figures P20.4 and P20.5). Keep this pitfall in mind whenever you see a lesion that is potentially extra-axial in either the interhemispheric fissure or sylvian fissure where it may be mistaken for an intra-axial mass (Figures P20.6–P20.11).

Correct answer: 2

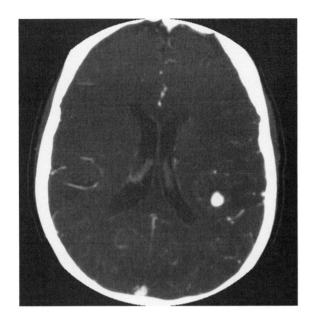

Figure P20.4

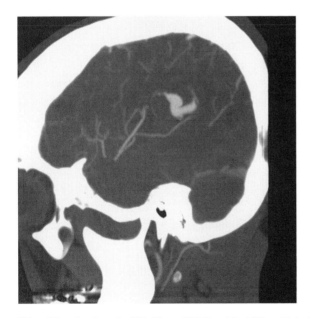

Figure P20.5

This axial section from the CTA (Figure P20.4) and the MIP sagittal reformat (Figure P20.5) demonstrate a serpentine, fusiform aneurysm of the left middle cerebral artery.

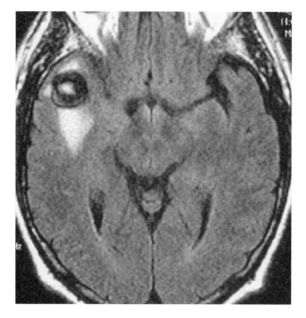

Figure P20.6

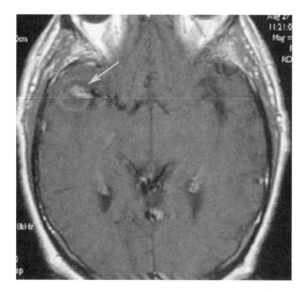

Figure P20.7

This patient with a right temporal mass was initially referred with the diagnosis of a brain tumor. This mass has a complete dark rim on T2WI (Figure P20.6) that at first glance suggests a cavernoma. The location at the MCA bifurcation and central enhancement (Figure P20.7, arrow), however, should at least suggest the diagnosis of aneurysm, which was confirmed on further imaging.

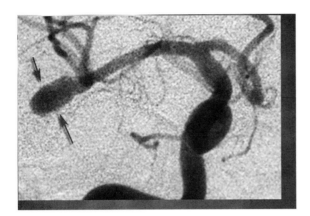

Figure P20.8 This image from the patient's cerebral angiogram demonstrates the aneurysm at the M1–2 junction of the right MCA (arrows). The angiogram, of course, only reveals the patent lumen. The actual aneurysm is larger, based on the MR appearance, where it appeared to be circumferentially filled with thrombus (Figure P20.6).

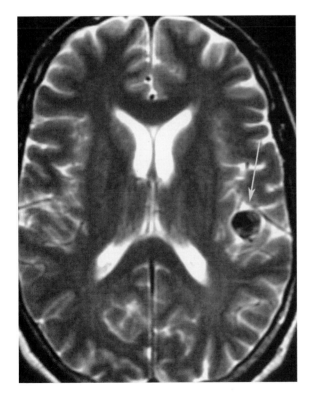

Figure P20.9

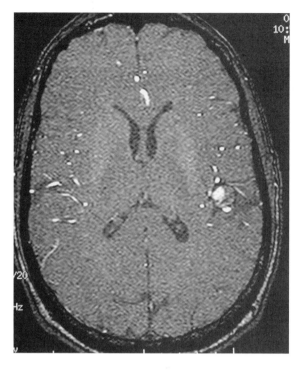

Figure P20.10

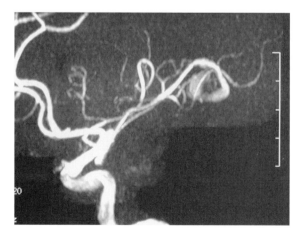

Figure P20.11

These images illustrate another example of a fusiform aneurysm of the MCA. It appears dark on the T2WI (Figure P20.9, arrow) due to both T2 shortening from thrombus and intravoxel dephasing from flow. Before considering any diagnosis, it is important to note that it resides in the sylvian fissure and therefore outside the brain. Magnetic resonance angiography (MRA) can be helpful whenever a vascular lesion is considered in the differential diagnosis of an intracranial lesion. This aneurysm is evident on the corresponding source image from the 3DTOF MRA scan (Figure P20.10) and the extent of the aneurysm lumen is evident on the MIP reconstruction (Figure P20.11).

Pitfall 21

This 54-year-old male presented with worsening headaches that began 2 days after finishing a 50-mile-long mountain bike ride. After reviewing the MIP from his 2D TOF MRA (Figure P21.1) and the sagittal T1WI through the region of his left transverse sinus (Figure P21.2), you think he has:

(1) acute thrombosis of the left transverse sinus.

(2) a sigmoid sinus occlusion with reversed flow in the transverse sinus.

(3) a normal but hypoplastic left transverse sinus.

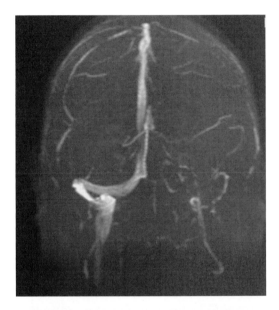

Figure P21.1

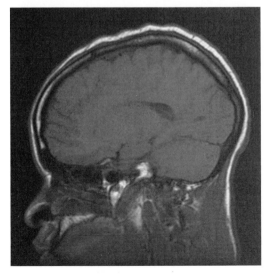

Figure P21.2

ASYMMETRY OF THE TRANSVERSE SINUSES AND MRV

This question of transverse sinus occlusion versus hypoplasia is a common one in clinical practice. A small dural sinus may be inapparent on MRV because of both limited resolution and slow flow velocity. There are clues that can help you to make the correct decision, however. First, it is important to acknowledge that asymmetry of the transverse sinuses is common. Second, spend some time reviewing the sagittal T1WI in the region of the absent sinus. If the sinus is visible and normal-sized or enlarged but with intermediate or increased signal, it may be occluded (Figure P21.3). If the sinus is inapparent on the T1WI and the occipital lobe meets the cerebellum, however, this favors the diagnosis of hypoplasia. Third, on the MRV, see if the jugular vein and the vein of Labbe are patent on the side of interest. There may be cases where you cannot be sure; in those instances, consider CT venogram (CTV; Figures P21.4 and P21.5).

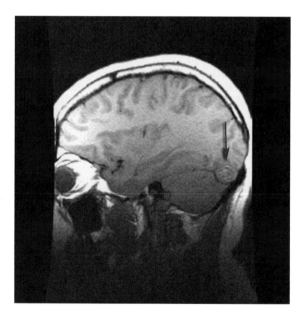

Figure P21.3 This sagittal scan from a patient with thrombosis of the transverse sinus demonstrates increased signal as well as expansion of the sinus (arrow).

Correct answer: 3

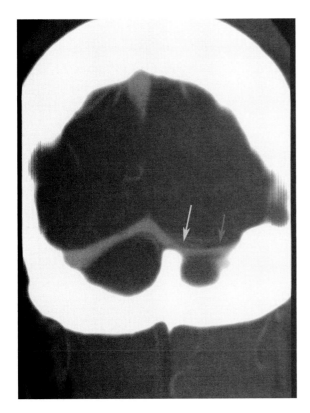

Figure P21.4

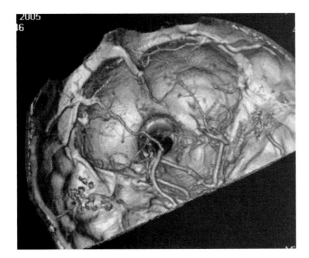

Figure P21.5

These are the multiplanar reconstruction (MPR) (Figure P21.4) and the surface model (Figure P21.5) from the computerized tomography venogram (CTV) of the patient depicted in Figure P21.1. They confirm the asymmetry of the transverse sinuses and at the same time show that the left transverse sinus is patent (Figure P21.4, arrows).

Pitfall 22

This recently married 35-year-old teacher presents with new headaches. His DWI (Figure P22.1) and axial enhanced T1WI (Figure P22.2) are provided. Your report would conclude that, based on the DWI and contrast scan, the juxtaventricular lesion:

(1) is a brain abscess.

(2) is a tumor.

(3) could be either.

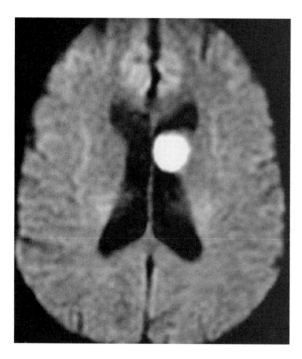

Figure P22.1

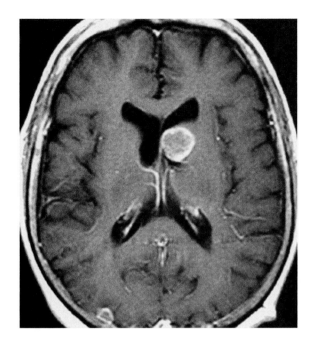

Figure P22.2

DIFFUSION MR OF BRAIN ABSCESS AND MIMICS

Moving protons may experience gradient reversals, which are intended to increase signal in *static* protons by reversing phase shifts, in a haphazard way and thereby accumulate unwelcome phase changes. These mixed-up protons cause intravoxel dephasing and thereby decreased signal on imaging, which explains why most arteries appear dark on all routine sequences.

Diffusion weighted imaging, on the other hand, makes a virtue of these signal-robbing phase shifts. By intentionally applying a balanced pair of gradients, the subsequent imaging will show that static protons provide more signal than mobile protons. In the case of DWI imaging, we are not talking about large movements, e.g. blood flow or pulsation of CSF, but rather about the unimaginably tiny movements of atoms and molecules.

In fact, these movements are so small that a single shot or echo planar scan is necessary in order to avoid having these movements overwhelmed by large movement of the tissues. Echo planar scanning is usually selected for DWI because it is an extremely fast imaging technique since all the phase encoding information is acquired in a single TR interval. Since there is a practical limit to how many lines of k-space can be filled in one TR interval, these scans use a relatively coarse matrix (128 x 128) compared with most other MR sequences that use 192 or 256 phase steps.

There are several artifacts that need to be considered when using this cheetah-fast technique among MR pulse sequences, however. Because of the method used for rapid filling of k-space, it is important

---

Correct answer: 2. This was a metastatic brain tumor and there is another in the right occipital lobe (P22.2).

to eliminate fat signal using chemical fat suppression; otherwise, large chemical shift artifacts will appear. Echo planar imaging, like many gradient echo techniques, is also very sensitive to inhomogeneities in the magnetic field. While one might go to great lengths to optimize the magnetic field with shim coils, the homogeneity of the magnetic field is sufficiently altered to be visible on echo planar scans by just placing a patient inside the scanner. At transitions between different structures, most evident at the skull base, there is enough distortion to obscure visualization of the anterior middle fossa in most patients.

The prototypical bright DWI lesion is the acute cerebral infarct. The cytotoxic edema that accompanies cell death is thought to result in the movement of extracellular water into the intracellular compartment, where its motion is restricted by the structures inside. This *restriction* of motion can be considered the cellular equivalent of walking barefoot through a dark room filled with chairs, tables, and sharp toys scattered about the floor compared with walking down a long, dark, obstacle-free hallway. The extra-cellular protons, once inside the infarcted brain cell, like the barefoot individual in the dark room, tend to move about less freely. This restricted motion results in those protons appearing bright on DWI because they would have experienced less dephasing after application of the balanced gradients than the protons that move freely about. This same effect is evident when imaging the pus in most bacterial brain abscesses (Figures P22.3 and P22.4)

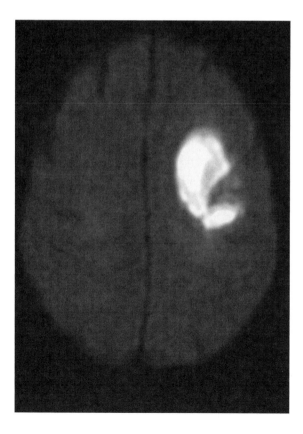

Figure P22.3

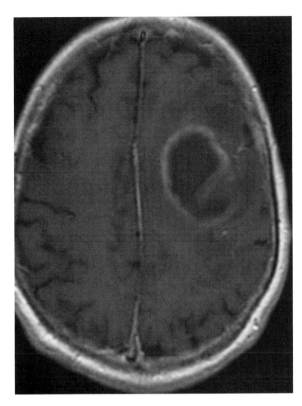

Figure P22.4

The diffusion scan (Figure P23.3) and the axial postcontrast T1WI (Figure P23.4) show typical features of a bacterial brain abscess i.e. rim enhancement and restricted diffusion in the center of the rim. This differs from the image P22.1 and P22.2 since there was the suggestion of central enhancement and the rim was also bright om DWI.

Because of the time necessary to apply the matching gradients, all clinical DWI images are a composite of diffusion and T2-weighted contrast. It is possible, however, to display just the calculated diffusion information in an image called an apparent diffusion coefficient map (ADC). This image is helpful and often necessary to determine whether a lesion is bright from restricted diffusion or from *shine through* of the T2-related signal (Figures P22.5 and P22.6).

Early on, it was thought that restricted diffusion within a ring enhancing mass might prove to be a unique diagnostic finding for brain abscess. Later, reports appeared of brain metastatic tumors or even primary tumors with a similar appearance, however. Their similarity in appearance may well be due to the similar physical properties, i.e., a central cavity filled with a viscous mix of protein, blood, or cellular debris. Keep this in mind when you see a ring enhancing mass that has high signal intensity on diffusion weighted imaging. Remember that the center, not the rim, of a brain abscess should show evidence of restricted diffusion. Careful attention to characterizing all parts of the lesion should be helpful. For example, there is the suggestion of central enhancement in P22.2 which is not expected with a mature abscess. While this distinction may be difficult in some cases, it is helpful just to be aware of this potential pitfall.

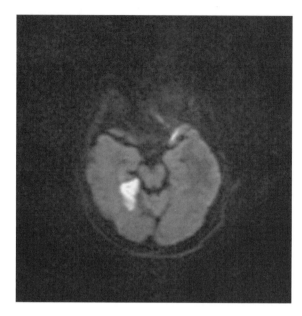

Figure P22.5

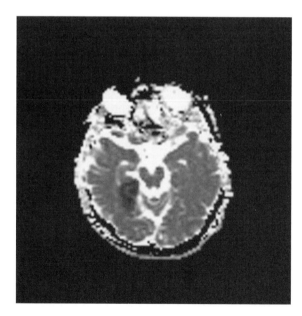

Figure P22.6

This diffusion-weighted scan (Figure P22.5) reveals a focal lesion in the right occipital lobe in a patient with an acute visual field cut. The ADC map (Figure P22.6) shows that this lesion is darker than normal brain, consistent with an acute infarct in the posterior cerebral territory with restricted diffusion.

Pitfall 23

This patient was referred for severe headaches with the indication "rule out vasculitis." On the basis of this DWI (Figure P23.1) and axial T1WI (Figure P23.2), you suspect that he has:

(1) occipital lobe embolic infarcts.

(2) a subdural hemorrhage.

(3) migraine headaches.

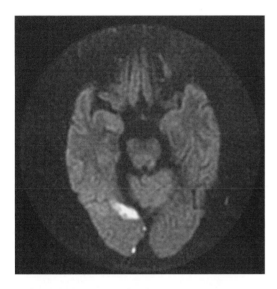

Figure P23.1

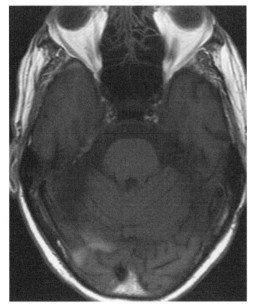

Figure P23.2

DIFFUSION AND THE EXTRA-AXIAL SPACE

This is a good example of the sometimes confusing appearance of subacute hemorrhage on DWI. You may have noticed how strongly the lesions in Figure 23.1 resembled the infarct in Figure P22.5, but the sagittal scan is very valuable here because it shows that the abnormality is actually located in the extra-axial space (Figure P23.3). Diffusion imaging of hemorrhage is confounded by the fact that the appearance of blood varies with age, since the diffusion, T2, and susceptibility effects all may contribute to DWI contrast (Figures P23.4 and P23.5). Because tumors, blood, and pus in the extra-axial space may show restricted diffusion it is essential to consider the clinical context (Figures P23.6–P23.11)

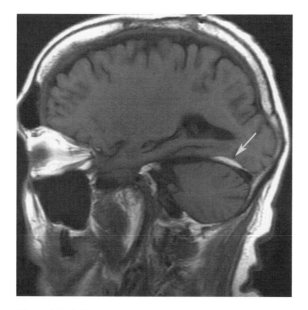

Figure P23.3 This sagittal T1WI shows linear high signal along the tentorium consistent with a subdural hemorrhage (Figure P23.3, arrow) that was volume averaged into the occipital lobe on both Figures P23.1 and P23.2.

Correct answer: 2

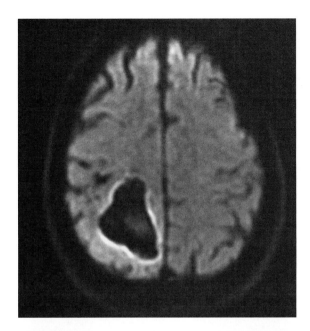

Figure P23.4

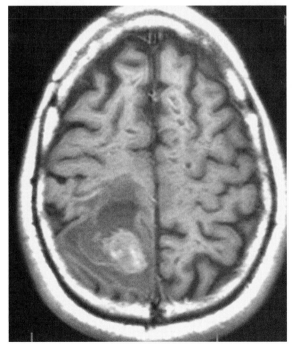

Figure P23.5

Here is a more acute brain hemorrhage seen on DWI (Figure P23.4) and axial T1WI (Figure P23.5). Note that this appears different than the subdural hemorrhage in Figure P23.1 and is nearly isointense on T1WI but has low signal on the DWI scan. The DWI appearance in this instance is due to signal loss from susceptibility effects of acute hemorrhage. Remember that this scan is an echo planar acquisition and, as such, is extremely sensitive to susceptibility effects.

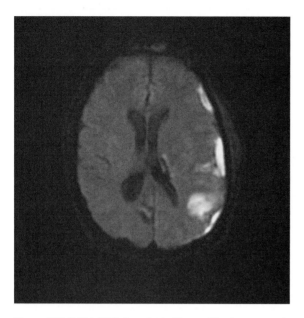

Figure P23.6 This DWI of a patient with an epidural empyema shows high signal in the left extra-axial space. Diffusion-weighted imaging is a very sensitive tool for the identification of pus because it has very restricted diffusion.

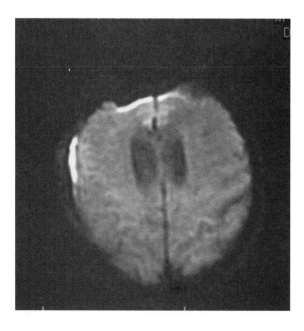

Figure P23.7

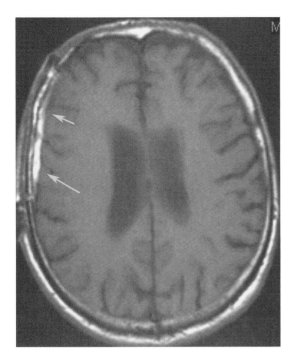

Figure P23.8

The DWI in Figure P23.7 is similar in appearance to Figure P23.6 but was obtained from a patient immediately after brain surgery. While there is high signal on DWI in the extra-axial space near the craniotomy, it is important to note that it appears bright on the axial T1WI (Figure P23.8, arrows) as well, and therefore would be most consistent with subacute blood which can also have restricted diffusion.

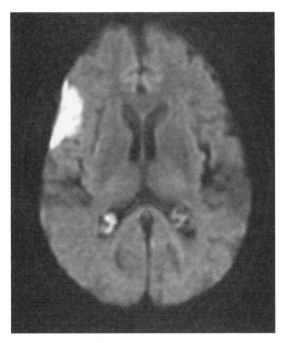

Figure P23.9

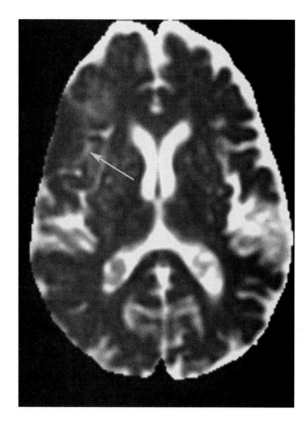

Figure P23.10

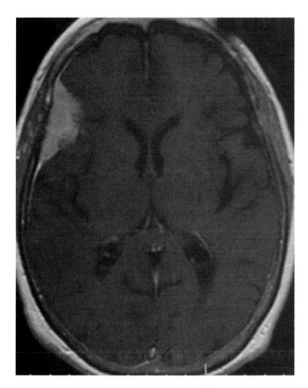

Figure P23.11

Figure P23.9 is a DWI of another patient with restricted diffusion in the extra-axial space. The ADC image (Figure P23.10) confirms that the high signal on DWI (arrow) represents restricted diffusion and not T2 shine through. The homogeneous enhancement on Figure P23.11 leads to the correct diagnosis of meningioma since empyema should only enhance peripherally. The restricted diffusion evident in many tumors, such as lymphoma, choroid plexus papilloma, medulloblastoma, and meningiomas, is thought to be due to dense cell packing with limitation to the free motion of water.

Pitfall 24

This 55-year-old male was brought to the emergency room after his wife found him lying unresponsive on the bathroom floor when she arrived home from work. He had felt ill at breakfast, with nausea, and had decided to stay home. The axial T1WI (Figure P24.1) and T2WI (Figure P24.2) at the level of the upper medulla are presented here. The neurology resident caring for him is concerned that he may have a brainstem infarct and asks, is the basilar artery open? On the basis of these images and history, you find that:

(1) there is slow flow in the basilar artery.

(2) The basilar artery is patent.

(3) The basilar artery is occluded.

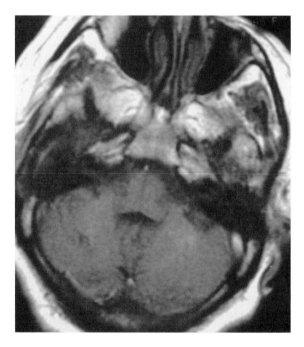

Figure P24.1

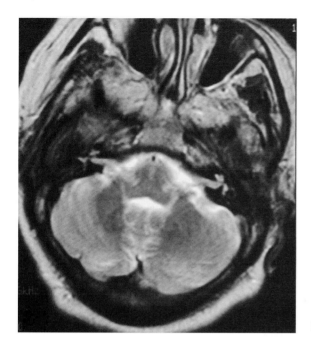

Figure P24.2

This case illustrates one of the difficulties of diagnosing an intravascular thrombus with MR. While the basilar artery appears normal on the T2WI, it is unusually bright on the T1WI. The key to making the correct diagnosis this case is to avoid discounting the T1WI appearance as entry slice or slow flow effects and at the same time to not mistake the low signal on T2WI as due to signal loss from intravoxel dephasing due to rapid flow. In this circumstance, the basilar artery low signal is due to the short T2 relaxation time of the acute thrombus (Figure P24.3). The sagittal T1WI is often helpful when the vertebral arteries appear bright on the axial scan. That is because on sagittal imaging inflow effects cannot explain high signal in a vessel, e.g. the basilar, that flows in a caudal to cranial direction (Figure P24.4).

Correct answer: 3

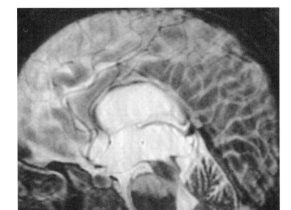

Figure P24.3 A sagittal T2WI obtained from this patient 2 days after the scans shown in Figure P24.1 and P14.2 shows a well-defined infarct of the upper pons from occlusion of pontine perforator arteries from this basilar artery thrombosis.

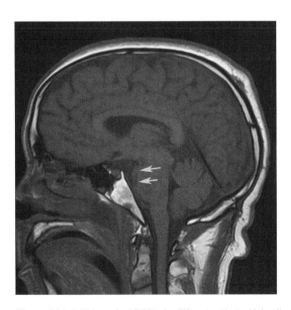

Figure P24.4 This sagittal T1WI of a different patient with basilar thrombosis shows intermediate signal in the basilar artery due to acute thrombus in the vessel (arrows).

Suggested Readings

Anzai Y, Ishikawa M, Shaw D, et al. Paramagnetic effect of supplemental oxygen on CSF hyperintensity on fluid-attenuated inversion recovery MR images. *AJNR.* 2004;25:274–279.

Edelman RR, Wielopolski P, Schmitt F. Echo-planar MR imaging. *Radiology.* 1994;192:600–612.

Hartmann M, Jansen O, Heiland S, et al. Restricted diffusion within ring enhancement is not pathognomonic for brain abscess. *AJNR.* 2001;22:1738–1742.

Hinman JM, Provenzale JM. Hypointense thrombus on T2-weighted MR imaging: a potential pitfall in the diagnosis of dural sinus thrombosis. *Eur J Radiol.* 2002;41:147–152.

Javan NG, Debnath J, Kumar A, et al. Oesophageal duplication cyst: an unusual cause of retrosternal pain and dysphagia in an adult. *Singapore Med J.* 2008;49(9):e242–e244.

Kinoshita T, Moritani T, Hiwatshi A, et al. Clinically silent choroids plexus cyst: evaluation by diffusion-weighted MRI. *Neuroradiology.* 2005;47:251–255.

Mamourian AC, Briggs RW. Appearance of Pantopaque on MR images. *Radiology.* 1986;158:457–460.

Moore KR, Harnsberger HR, Shelton C, et al. "Leave me alone" lesions of the petrous apex. *AJNR.* 1998;19:733–738.

Pastel DA, Mamourian AC, Duhaime AC. Internal structure in pineal cysts on high-resolution magnetic resonance imaging: not a sign of malignancy. *J Neurosurg Pediatrics.* 2009;4:81–84.

Salzman KL, Osborn AG, House P, et al. Giant tumefactive perivascular spaces. *AJNR.* 2005;26:298–305.

VandeVyver V, Lemmerling M, Foer BD, et al. Arachnoid granulations of the posterior temporal bone wall: imaging appearance and differential diagnosis. *AJNR.* 2007;28:610–612.

4 TEN PUZZLERS

You can use these 10 test cases to test your acumen with MR. If you choose to test yourself before reading the book, don't feel badly if you don't nail all 10. This should provide motivation to carefully read the rest of the book. If you get them all, well I hope you can still can find some wisdom within these pages.

Test Case 1

The coronal (Figure C1.1) and axial (Figure C1.2) T2WI scans demonstrate a complex left hemi-spheric brain tumor. What is your diagnosis?

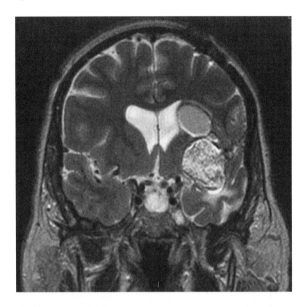

Figure C1.1

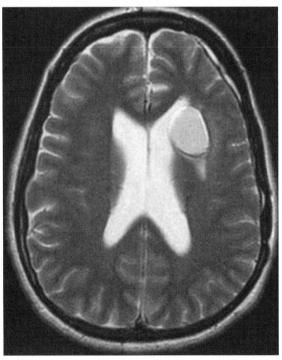

Figure C1.2

While the presence of a chemical shift artifact in this case suggests the possibilities of both lipoma and dermoid, the complex appearance of the mass and the off-midline location favor the diagnosis of dermoid. The appearance of the T1WI (Figure C1.3), with droplets of fat along the sylvian fissure and in the right ventricle, and the CT (Figure C1.4) establishes the diagnosis of a ruptured dermoid.

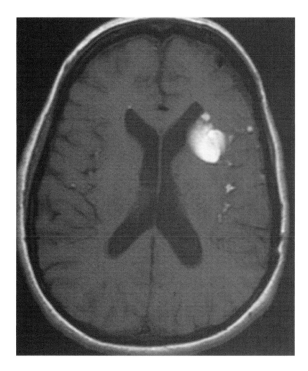

Figure C1.3 This axial T1WI also shows short T1 material in the subarachnoid space consistent with a ruptured dermoid.

Correct diagnosis: Intracranial Dermoid.

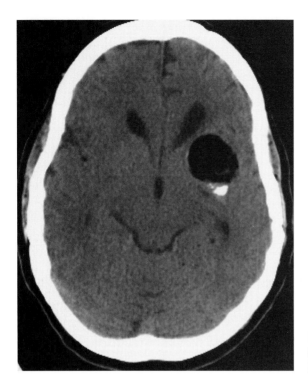

Figure C1.4 This axial section is from the CT scan from the same patient. Note the low attenuation compatible with fat and high attenuation from calcification in this dermoid.

Test Case 2

This MR scan of a patient with a family history of aneurysm and headaches includes T2WI (Figures C2.1 and C2.2), 3D TOF (Figures C2.3 and C2.4), and T2*Gradient Echo (Figure C2.5).

How would you explain the appearance of the left hemispheric lesion?

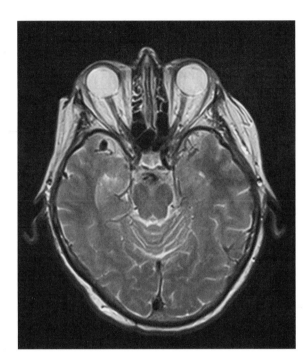

Figure C2.1

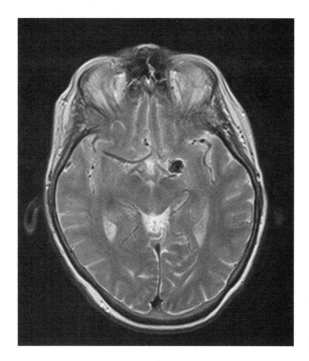

Figure C2.2

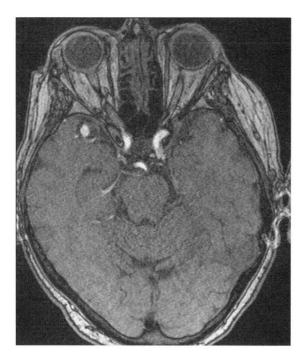

Figure C2.3

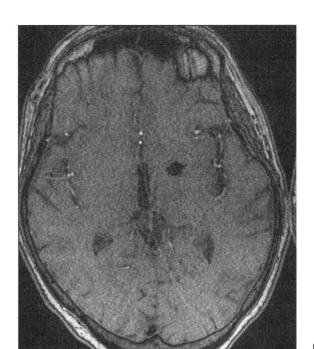

Figure C2.4

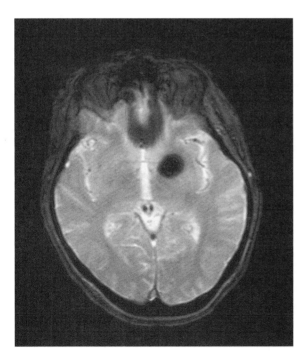

Figure C2.5

The patient has two aneurysms, one at the right M1–2 junction and one at the left carotid apex. No flow is evident on the 3D TOF, however, in the left-sided aneurysm, and a large susceptibility artifact is apparent on the gradient echo scan (Figure C2.5). While you may wonder if this indicates that this aneurysm is thrombosed, the size of the susceptibility artifact on the gradient echo scan is too large for just thrombus. In fact, the signal drop out is the result of metal artifact from previous treatment with coils (Figure C2.6). The small size of the artifact on the 3D TOF source image (Figure C2.4) argues against previous treatment with an aneurysm clip since one would expect to see a larger and asymmetric susceptibility artifact (see Artifact 15 in Chapter 2). The platinum coils used for aneurysm treatment cause so little artifact on MR that MRA is commonly used for follow-up imaging to determine if there is recanalization of the aneurysm lumen.

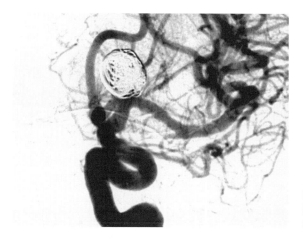

Figure C2.6 Posttreatment digital subtraction angiography DSA image demonstrating the coil mass in a carotid apex aneurysm.

Correct answer: Postcoiling of a carotid terminus aneurysm and an untreated right middle cerebral artery aneurysm.

Test Case 3

These images, axial FLAIR (Figure C3.1), T1WI (Figure C3.2), and axial T1WI with contrast (Figure C3.3), were obtained in a young patient who was suspected of having sarcoidosis based on a lung biopsy. What is your diagnosis?

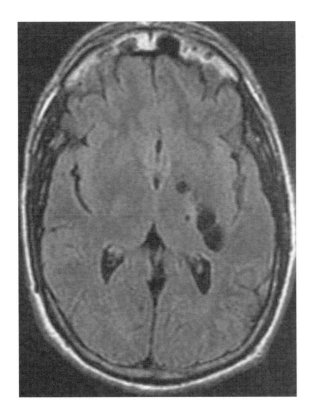

Figure C3.1

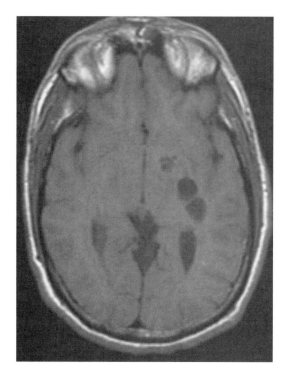

Figure C3.2

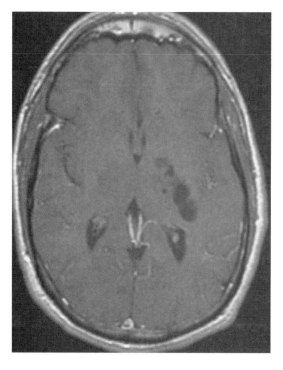

Figure C3.3

The absence of enhancement or any significant abnormal signal on the FLAIR scan supports the diagnosis that these are benign, dilated CSF cysts (see Pitfall 20 in Chapter 3).

Correct answer: Tumefactive perivascular spaces.

Test Case 4

On the basis of this single T1WI of a patient with severe headaches 1 week postpartum (Figure C4.1), what is your diagnosis?

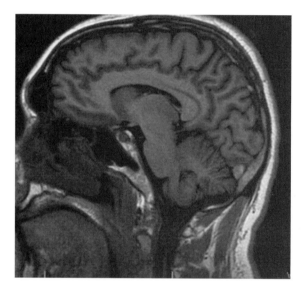

Figure C4.1

The high signal in the transverse sinus could mean that it was open and bright as a result of entry slice effect if the ipsilateral sigmoid sinus was occluded and flow was reversed. Since flow in the transverse sinus goes medial to lateral, you should not expect to see flow-related enhancement normally. In this case the occluded transverse sinus is confirmed on the phase contrast MR venogram (MRV) since no flow is evident (Figure C4.2) this represents T1 shortening due to subacute thrombus. When you see high signal in a normal size transverse sinus, consider venous occlusion.

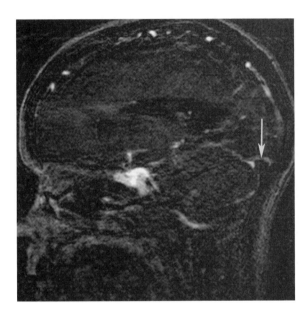

Figure C4.2 The sagittal phase contrast MRV shows no evidence of flow in the abnormal transverse sinus (arrow), although flow in the cortical veins and cavernous sinus is apparent.

Correct answer: Transverse sinus occlusion.

Test Case 5

This 26-year-old professional skier presented with new knee pain. Her MR scan demonstrated increased signal in the bone marrow on the postcontrast T1WI sagittal scan (Figure C5.1). Her STIR (Figure C5.2) and T1WI (Figure C5.3) scans are provided. What is your diagnosis?

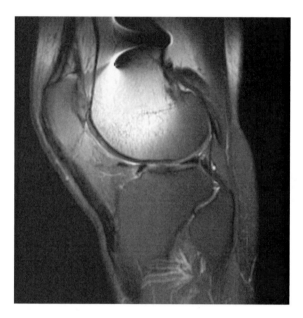

Figure C5.1

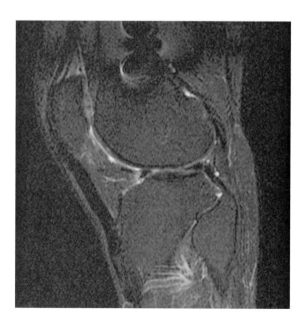

Figure C5.2

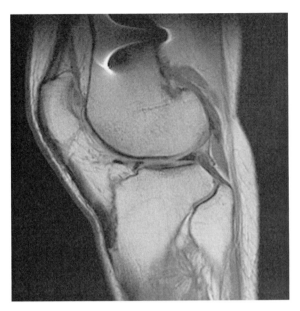

Figure C5.3

The sagittal STIR (Figure C5.2) and T1WI (Figure C5.3) are available at the same location as C5.1 for comparison. (Images provided by Douglas Goodwin, MD, Dartmouth-Hitchcock Medical Center, Lebanon, NH.)

Since chemical fat suppression requires accurate delivery of the initial RF pulse tuned to the frequency of fat, anything that distorts the magnetic field may interfere with the quality of the fat suppression. The normal appearance on STIR, and serpiginous high- and low-signal artifacts in the distal femur, indicate that the marrow findings on the fat-suppressed T1WI (Figure C5.1) are due to metal artifact causing incomplete fat suppression (see Artifact 9).

Correct answer: Incomplete fat saturation due to distortion arising from metal in the femur s/p prior ACL repair.

Test Case 6

An axial T1WI of the pelvis is available (Figure C6.1). One of the other two images is a STIR image of the same patient. Is it Figure C6.2 or Figure C6.3? Hint: Do you think this patient has an endometrioma or a dermoid?

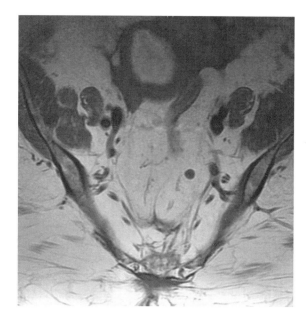

Figure C6.1

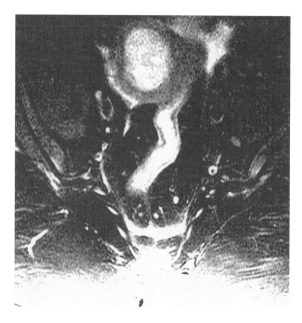

Figure C6.2

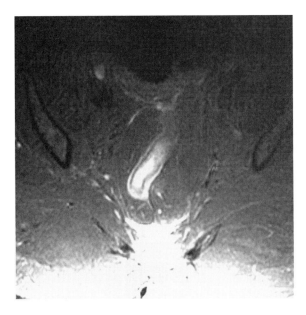

Figure C6.3

The tipoff in this case is the rounded mass in the midline that is bright on only two of the three pulse sequences. We know it has some T1 shortening based on the initial T1WI. In Figure C6.2 it is still bright, while the fat is now dark. This suggests that it is a fat-suppressed T2WI since the bowel contents and pelvic fluid are both bright. Since the mass does not suppress, that fact argues against a dermoid because fat in a dermoid would be expected to suppress as well. That leaves the STIR image as Figure C6.3, and the T1 shortening within the mass must be due to blood products rather than fat. Since STIR will suppress any short T1 tissue, the pelvic fat and the hemorrhagic cyst both appear dark in Figure C6.3.

Correct answer: Figure C6.3 is the STIR scan.

Test Case 7

This 62-year-old female presents with diminished vision in the left eye. The axial (Figure C7.1) and coronal (Figure C7.2) TIWI, both with fat suppression and IV contrast, show high signal in the left orbit. What is your diagnosis?

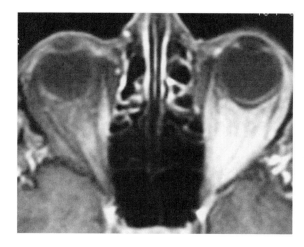

Figure C7.1

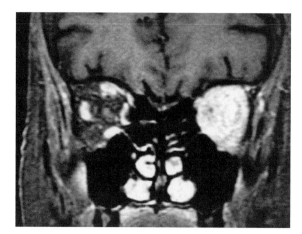

Figure C7.2

I wanted to get your attention if you were expecting an artifact. While you should consider the possibility of incomplete fat suppression, there is no evidence of metal distortion anywhere on these images. In this case, the coronal unenhanced T1WI (Figure C7.3), where one would not expect to see effects of metal distortion, demonstrates the left orbital tumor infiltrating or displacing the orbital fat.

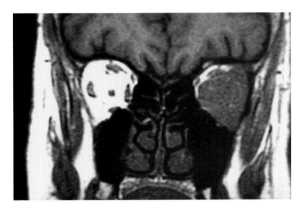

Figure C7.3

Correct answer: Left eye tumor, which proved to be lymphoma.

Test Case 8

This patient presented with low back pain, and an MR scan was requested. The scout view was obtained using a gradient echo technique. You notice something abnormal when you review the scout view (Figure C8.1), which is your (good) habit. What is wrong with this scout view?

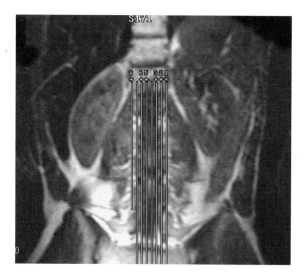

Figure C8.1

This patient had unrecognized hemochromatosis that was identified on this scout view. The follow-up examination of the liver demonstrated low signal due to rapid dephasing of the hydrogen protons characteristic of this condition (Figure C8.2). The iron distributed throughout the liver shortens the T2* relaxation time to the point where it difficult to recover signal on a T2 or gradient echo scan. Note the normal appearance of the spleen, indicating that this is not a case of hemosiderosis.

There is a family of contrast agents that use iron effects to suppress signal from normal liver in order to highlight tumors. Because the particles of iron in these agents have magnetic properties somewhere between ferromagnetism and paramagnetism, this behavior is called *superparamagnetism*.

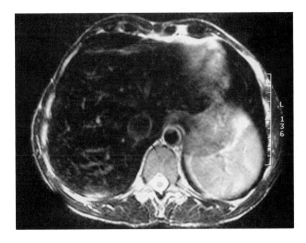

Figure C8.2 This axial T2WI (note the CSF) shows a very dark liver but a normal spleen typical of iron deposition from hemochromatosis. The magnetic properties of iron cause rapid dephasing of the liver protons (short T2 relaxation time) and thereby signal loss on this T2WI.

Correct answer: Unusually dark liver due to hemochromatosis.

Test Case 9

Figure C9.1 is the 2D TOF MRA from an 18-year-old patient with new neck pain and dizziness. What is your diagnosis?

  (1) normal.

  (2) carotid dissection.

  (3) early atherosclerosis.

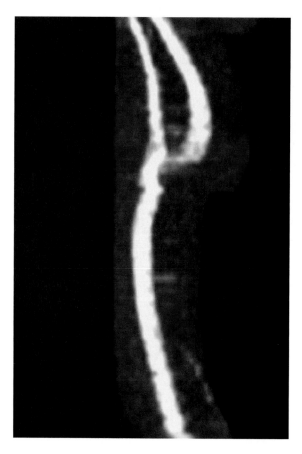

Figure C9.1

The 2D TOF scan (Figure C9.1) demonstrates a signal void in the posterior carotid bulb. While this could be due to atherosclerosis in a different scenario, in this young patient it is more likely to be the result of the recirculation of flow in a normal carotid bulb. Since 2D TOF imaging suppresses all caudal flow to eliminate the signal from veins, the saturation band will also suppress caudal arterial flow. The contrast MRA scan, obtained immediately after the 2D TOF exam, revealed a normal contour of the bulb in this case (Figure C9.2).

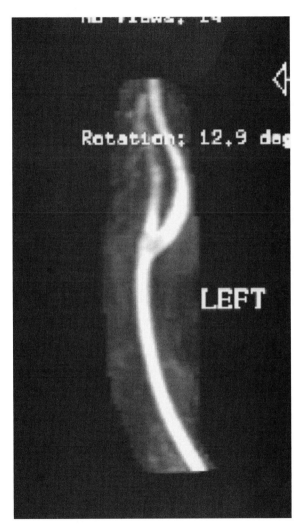

Figure C9.2

Correct answer: Normal.

Test Case 10

This patient, with persistent neck pain and a history of smoking, had an MR scan with the indication "rule out malignancy." The sagittal T1WI through the left internal jugular vein (Figure C10.1) shows striking high signal compared with the normal flow void seen on the sagittal T1WI through the right internal jugular vein (Figure C10.2). This asymmetry is evident on the axial T2WI as well (Figure C10.3). Perhaps this is a thrombus associated abnormal coagulation due to malignancy? What is your diagnosis? (Hint: consider the background noise.)

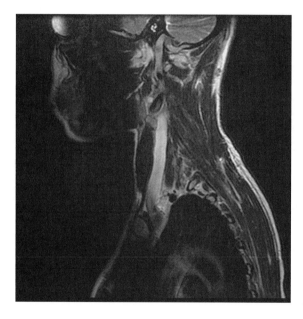

Figure C10.1

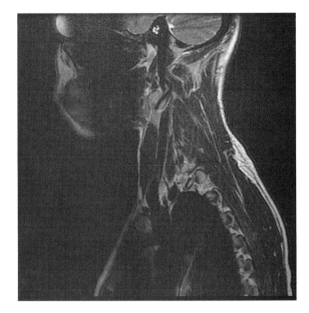

Figure C10.2

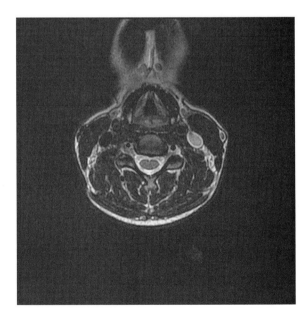

Figure C10.3

As you look for the imaging features of either thrombus or slow flow in this case, it is helpful to consider that the anatomy of the left jugular is not symmetric with the right jugular. The right jugular joins with the subclavian vein before draining directly into the superior vena cava via a short innominate vein. The left innominate vein, which is nearly twice as long as the right, must cross the midline. Slow flow, as well as reversed flow, in the left jugular vein can be secondary to compression of this left innominate vein by the aorta as the vein passes under the sternum. It is for this reason that it is best to always inject contrast into a right arm vein whenever possible for both CTA and MRA in order to avoid reflux up the left jugular. The key to establishing the presence of flow in this case is the observation of a vascular ghost on the axial image (Figure C10.4) since that would not be expected with an occluded vessel.

> Correct answer: Slow flow in the left jugular vein, most likely from compression of the innominate vein by an ectatic aorta.

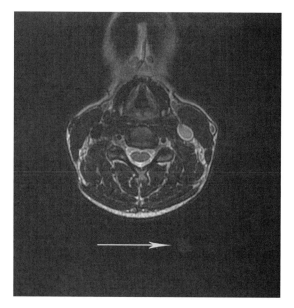

Figure C10.4

Suggested Reading

Tanaka T, Uemura K, Takahashi M, et al. Compression of the left brachiocephalic vein: cause of high signal intensity of the left sigmoid sinus and internal jugular vein on MR images. *Radiology.* 1993;188:355–361.

INDEX

	DATE DUE		